Aesthetic Breast Augmentation Revision Surgery

Roy de Vita

Editor

Aesthetic Breast Augmentation Revision Surgery

From Problem to Solution

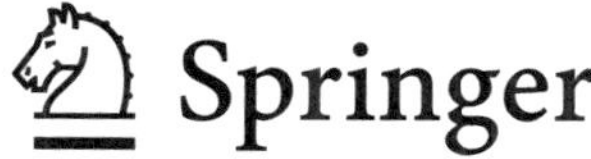 Springer

Editor
Roy de Vita
Department of Plastic Surgery
National Institute for Cancer, "Regina Elena"
Rome, Italy

ISBN 978-3-030-86795-9   ISBN 978-3-030-86793-5   (eBook)
https://doi.org/10.1007/978-3-030-86793-5

This Springer imprint is published by the registered company Springer Nature Switzerland AG
The registered company address is: Gewerbestrasse 11, 6330 Cham, Switzerland

Preface

Writing a skillful yet compact guide is not an easy undertaking, but with this volume titled Aesthetic Breast Augmentation Revision Surgery: From Problem to Solution we believe in having succeeded in creating an essentially practical work which indicates corrective interventions and, according to the case at hand, helps choosing the most suitable technical option.

The journey from the first idea to its publication was a long one, and thanks to my co-worker Dr. E.M. Buccheri and his unwavering commitment, the work of all involved was steered to safe haven. The chapters are written by well-renowned plastic surgeons from all around the world, offering a comprehensive overview of the complex and ample topic of secondary aesthetic breast surgery.

The book includes eight chapters, covering subjects as the algorithm for secondary breast surgeries in capsular contracture treatment, and how to deal with the issues of double bubble deformity or implant rotation, to the convoluted management of inframammary fold, the correction of symmastia, up to addressing the need for implant substitution caused by implant infection, exposure, or rupture.

We believe that its very specific topic makes this volume a unique contribution to the field; thoroughly illustrated, it will be essential reading not only for plastic surgeons—whose work goes beyond borders of different surgical specializations—but for all surgeons who wish to be updated on the most current techniques and interested in deepening their understanding of aesthetic breast surgery.

Rome, Italy

October 2021

Roy de Vita

Acknowledgments

This book could not have reached publication without the support of Springer's editorial and production team. A very grateful and special word of thanks goes to the excellent work of my colleague and assistant Doctor Ernesto Maria Buccheri, whose steadfast dedication and passion have supported me in this publication journey.

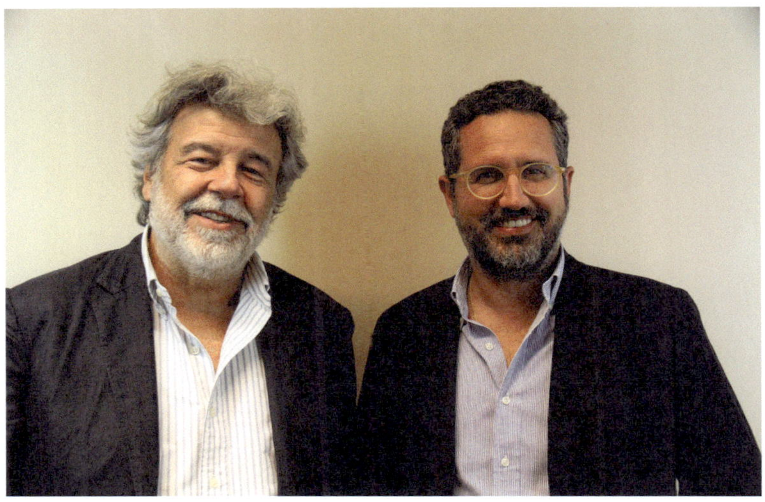

Contents

Algorithm for Secondary Aesthetic Breast Surgery

Patrick Mallucci and Giovanni Bistoni

1   Introduction

Breast augmentation is the most popularly carried out procedure in aesthetic surgery worldwide. Approximately 80,000 operations are carried out in the US alone on a yearly basis. Whilst both implant manufacturing and the process of breast augmentation have vastly improved over the past six decades, complication rates remain high. The reasons for complications are multifactorial: they include iatrogenic causes such as poor implant selection, poor surgical technique, and poor process including neglected post-operative care. Other causes are related to the implants themselves and their inherent deficiencies. Patient anatomy whether it be in primary or secondary situations also plays an important part in determining outcome and potential complications. The most comprehensive overview of implant performance and complication rates has been derived from the core studies with Allergan and Mentor implants [1]. There are numerous other studies looking at complications and outcomes from single surgeon or single centre units defining key determinants relating to poor outcome [2–5].

In order to be able to correct poor outcome, it is important to be able to define its nature. Poor outcome may simply relate to 'look' or dissatisfaction thereof. The latter may relate to implant malposition, an unidentified or recurrent ptosis, dissatisfaction with size or a particular type of appearance, i.e. too fake or too natural. It may relate to unmet expectations, perhaps unrealistic at the outset. Other complications might be more tangible: an implant rupture, capsular contracture, infection, and extrusion. The overlay of anatomy on all of these situations is also critical. Those with poor soft tissues, thin skin, little native breast tissue, multiple scars,

P. Mallucci (✉)
Mallucci London, London, UK
e-mail: pm@mallucci-london.com

G. Bistoni
Plastic Surgery Unit, Department of Surgery, Sapienza University of Rome, Rome, Italy

© Springer Nature Switzerland AG 2022
R. de Vita (ed.), *Aesthetic Breast Augmentation Revision Surgery*,
https://doi.org/10.1007/978-3-030-86793-5_1

multiple past procedures, as well as little body fat all pose significant reconstructive challenges, with higher complication rates. As with all complications, the best form of treatment is prevention in the first instance. Making the sensible choice at the outset is the key. It is critical that the patient is led by the surgeon and not vice versa, patients will often not understand the limitations of their own anatomy on implant selection, the concept of 'it's not what you want, it's what you can have' is a reflection of this point. Today's approach to breast augmentation should follow the principles of tissue-based planning, where the patient's anatomy is the determining factor around implant choice. Many methods have been described in the literature to help this process, such as the ICE principle [6], the AK method described by Heden [7], the High 5 by Tebbets and Adams [8], and the Y number of del Yerro [9]. Whilst they all differ to some extent, they all attempt to match implant selection to the soft tissue characteristics of the breast, thereby adhering to very similar principles.

Fundamental to all aesthetic surgery is a baseline or norm which serves as a framework around which to plan not only in primary surgery, but also perhaps even more importantly for secondary corrective procedures. In the breast, the aesthetic ideals have been well characterised by the author, with four fundamental parameters as markers for attractiveness: the 45:55 volume distribution between the upper and the lower pole (i.e. the lower pole always slightly fuller than the upper pole), a skyward pointing nipple, a tight convex curve to the lower pole with adequate tension to elevate it off the upper abdomen, and a natural upper pole slope—straight line or very mildly concave [10, 11].

These parameters are especially important when analysing poor outcomes, in order to be able to make the correct decisions in order to be able to restore these parameters to recreate a positive outcome.

2 Causes of Secondary Surgery

In order to maximise outcome and minimise the likelihood of complications and re-operation, the principles for planning focus on several points: patient selection, patient education, pre-operative planning and implant selection, precise surgical technique, and a defined process for post-operative care [4]. These principles highlight the fact that prevention of complications in the first instance is the most effective way to reduce re-operation rates. As previously stated, the causes for re-operation are multifactorial. Examples include the selection of oversized implants, failure to optimise soft tissue cover over the implant, traumatic pocket dissection leading to subclinical haematoma in the peri-implant space, excessive handling of the breast implant, and failure to maintain a strictly aseptic surgical environment. Steps to avoid this have been clearly laid out in the 14-point plan of Adams et al. [12].

Surgical complications in breast implant surgery could also be classified as pre- and intra-operative complications as well as early and late post-operative complications. Pre-operative and intra-operative complications derive from poor planning (wrong implant selection, wrong choice of the surgical access, incorrect surgical plane) or poor surgical technique (over-dissection of the implant pocket, implant malpositioning, excessive bleeding). Early post-operative complications include haematoma, seroma, infection, implant malposition and pain. Late post-operative complications include infection, seroma, capsular contracture, excessive pectoral animation, implant visibility, implant malposition (descent, double bubble, waterfall deformity), implant rippling, wrinkling and palpability, implant rupture, symmastia, poor scar healing or scar hypertrophy [13]. However, it has to be taken into account that some re-operations are inherently unavoidable and may relate to other patient factors such as pregnancy, weight fluctuations, natural ageing, or hormonal changes within the breast.

The best evidence relating to silicone gel-filled breast implants derives from the US Food and Drug Administration (FDA) core studies—10-year follow-up data regarding Natrelle 410 anatomical form-stable silicone-filled breast implants (Allergan Inc., Irvine, California) used in aesthetic and reconstructive breast surgery [14]. The Allergan core study investigated the safety and effectiveness of Natrelle 410 breast implants reporting complications and re-operation rates, reporting the cumulative risk of a subject experiencing an adverse event at any time during the investigation period (10 years). Capsular contracture rates (Baker scale grades III and IV) at 10-year follow-up were 9.2% for augmentation and 14.5% for reconstruction. The confirmed rupture rate was 9.4% without any report of extracapsular silicone gel migration. Other major complications (>5%) were implant malposition (4.7% for augmentation) and asymmetry (6.9%). The seroma rate was 1.6% for augmentation subjects, 0.6% occurring more than 1 year after implantation (late seroma). A single case of breast implant-associated anaplastic large cell lymphoma (BIA-ALCL) was reported.

The 410 Allergan core study concluded that the most commonly reported complication in breast implant surgery is capsular contracture, the risk of this complication increasing over time, even though capsular contracture rates being lower than those observed in the Natrelle round gel (fourth generation) core study, mostly including smooth implants (56.2%) [15]

Similarly the 6-year data about the form-stable Mentor Contour Profile Gel (CPG) implants (Mentor Worldwide LLC, Santa Barbara, California) showed lower contracture rates for the CPG implants when compared with predominantly smooth-surface round gel breast implants [16, 17]. The 10-year data also show a very low rate of implant rippling or wrinkling (0.9% for augmentation, 6.2% for reconstruction).

In summary, the most common indications for secondary surgery are size change, capsular contracture, implant malposition, and implant rupture and these may be classified into three categories: to the surgical procedure, to soft tissue changes and related to the implant [4] (Table 1).

Table 1 Causes of secondary breast implant surgery

Related to the operation
– Selection of incorrect procedure (implant versus mastopexy)
– Postsurgical fluid collection
– Selection of incorrect implant
– Failure to optimise soft tissue cover
– Excessively traumatic pocket dissection
– Overdissection/underdissection of the pocket
– Iatrogenic implant damage
– Overrelease/underrelease of muscle
– Suboptimal surgical instrumentation
Related to soft tissue changes
– Elongation of the lower pole
– Atrophy of tissue
– Stretching and thinning of tissue
– Breast tissue/glandular hypertrophy
– Development of ptosis
Related to the implant
– Rupture
– Malposition
– Rotation
– Capsular contracture
– Malposition
– Rippling
– Palpability
– Implant edge visibility

3 Problem Solving Algorithm

In order to simplify the process of problem solving only two fundamental aspects need to be considered in corrective surgery: the soft tissue component and the implant. These are the only elements that are correctable either on their own or collectively. They also have to be considered on the back of the 45:55 template. The following are a list of changeable elements in either the soft tissues or the implant selection:

3.1 Soft Tissue Component

The plane.
Embellishment with fat.
Soft tissue manipulation mastopexy/tightening/reduction.
Introduction of extraneous support—Mesh/ADM.

3.2 The Implant

Size—downsize/upsize.
Shape—round/anatomical.
Gel—softer, firmer, B-lite.
Texture—smooth, micro/macro textured, polyurethane.
These elements will be considered in more depth.

4 The Soft Tissue Components

4.1 The Plane

This may be a relatively straightforward problem where, for example, a visible implant lying in the subglandular plane may benefit from a plane change to a submuscular plane (dual plane) in order to achieve better cover.

Occasionally a plane change in the opposite direction may be necessary, i.e. from subpectoral to subglandular as, for example, in the case of a double bubble or where there is excessive animation deformity.

A 'third' space exists as a neo-subpectoral pocket described by Maxwell, in which implants already in the subpectoral plane can be placed into a neopocket by creating a space between the anterior capsule adherent to the posterior surface of the pectoralis major by peeling it off the muscle and suturing it to the posterior capsule on the chest wall [18]. This is useful when placing anatomical implants into a breast where the implants have been previously placed in subpectoral pocket in order to minimise the risk of rotation or to determine new boundaries to limit the pocket as in a correction of a symmastia.

4.2 Soft Tissue Manipulation—e.g. Mastopexy

It is not uncommon for an individual to present with dissatisfaction around the appearance of the breasts. Often an untreated or unrecognised ptosis or tissue laxity is not addressed at the original surgery, sometimes it is the patient who has insisted she doesn't want scars or the surgeon who claims he/she can obtain a good result without scars. Therefore, the addition of a mastopexy to correct secondary cases is common, whether this be a lesser circumareolar procedure or a more complete inverted T mastopexy.

Also, in secondary surgery where downsizing of the pre-existing implant is common, secondary mastopexy is often required as a tailoring procedure around the smaller implant with tightening and lifting as required.

The inverted T gives a much more comprehensive re-shaping than the simpler procedures and it is important to understand that mastopexy is not simply about nipple elevation but about re-organisation of the breast as a whole. It was stipulated earlier in the chapter the importance of using the 45:55 as a framework concept around which to plan for secondary cases where form and shape are often highly distorted.

4.3   Fat Transfer

Fat transfer is a powerful tool in the case of secondary surgery. It can be used in many forms and for several indications. Examples include the correction of asymmetries, softening of cleavage gaps, as cover for implant visibility, and correction of specific defects. Patient expectation has to be managed with respect to the use of fat transfer and its survival. On average, patients are advised that approximately 50% of injected fat will survive, they are therefore counselled regarding the possible need to repeat the procedure after some months in order to add a further layer should this be required. Management of the capsule in patients having fat transfer is important especially where tissues are extremely thin. The presence of the capsule can be important as a defined structure for the containment of fat superficial to the implant. Fat can also be used as a preparatory step in the process of restoration. In other words, prior to the insertion of the implant it can be layered into the breast in preparation for placement at a later date once the soft tissue conditions have improved as a result of the fat transfer.

4.4   Mesh/ADM

There are occasions where extraneous assistance is required. In patients who are extremely thin with no fat available, or where the soft tissue quality or skin conditions are particularly poor, local manoeuvres to accommodate implants such as capsulorrhaphies and the like might be deemed insufficient. The use of ADMs in both reconstructive and aesthetic breast surgery is well documented. As well as a supporting role, their minimal thickness may have some use in providing implant cover in desperate situations where nil else is available. However, the cost of ADMs is often prohibitive in the self-pay market, and their benefits have to be balanced against cost.

The advent of various Meshes has been significant in aesthetic breast surgery. Not only are they more affordable, but their ease of use, wide range of indications, and lower complication rates make them a very attractive alternative to ADMs. The author has extensive experience with the use of GalaFlex mesh—P4HB, a biologically derived, biodegradable monofilament polymer. The mesh is broken down over a 2-year period and converted to collagen which in itself carries tensile strength beyond the life of the mesh.

The mesh is incorporated extremely rapidly into the tissues. It is not associated with negative complications such as red breast syndrome or seromas as seem with

ADMs and is an extremely useful adjunct in difficult secondary cases for implant malposition and synmastia.

5 The Implant—Changeable Elements

As mentioned above, there are many aspects of an implant that can be changed. A comprehensive understanding of how different elements of implant characteristics can be of benefit in difficult situations is essential in order to undertake complex revisional surgery.

5.1 Implant Volume—Down Size/Upsize

This is self-explanatory. Volume increase or decrease can be beneficial according to the situation in hand. In most cases the problem is that the implant is too big; this leads to secondary complications such as edge visibility, rippling, unnatural contours, malposition such as bottoming out, tissue thinning, ptosis and double bubble. In such cases downsizing is often part of the solution. This may be accompanied by secondary procedures such as mastopexy and/or fat transfer.

On occasion, underfilling can be a problem and therefore a moderate increase in size may be beneficial.

5.2 Implant Shape

It is very important to understand the difference between anatomic and round implants.

Anatomical implants can be changed in three dimensions independently of each other, the height, the width and the projection. Round implants can only be changed in two dimensions. This versatility can be extremely useful when dealing with complex asymmetries either as primary problems or as secondary complications.

The other key difference between the devices is the volume distribution and the maximum point of projection. The low projection point of the anatomical implant allows for an upward rotation of the NAC and filling of the lower pole of the breast in cases of tissue laxity such as iatrogenic waterfall deformities or pseudoptotic breasts.

Change from one shape to another can solve many issues of volume maldistribution especially where there is excessive upper pole volume. The latter often leads to downward pointing nipples because of the high projection point of the pre-existing round implants. A simple change in shape from round to anatomical can easily solve the matter.

Occasionally change from anatomical to round implant is indicated, especially for recurrent rotation or where the anatomy favours the round implant.

5.3 Implant Texture/Surface

The subject of implant texture is a highly pertinent one especially in this age of BIA-ALCL. Whilst an in-depth discussion about texture and ALCL is beyond the remit of this chapter, it is important to understand that to have no texture (only smooth) essentially means eliminating anatomical implants from use. The author does not believe this to be appropriate at this time given the rarity of the condition. As has been illustrated anatomical implants confer certain advantages that round implants are unable to match due to their shape difference. To date, apart from France, texture has not been banned in Europe and a large variety of surfaces are available for use, from smooth to micro/macro textures and polyurethane. The latter is particularly useful in secondary surgeries especially for anatomically shaped implants to prevent rotation. The Introduction of anatomical implants into previously dissected implant pockets which lack stability and are no longer tailor made to the newly selected implants lead to a high incidence of implant rotation. A change of plane can help to create a 'new' pocket, e.g. from subglandular to a subpectoral pocket, or from a subpectoral pocket to a neo-subpectoral pocket; however, pocket stability is difficult to control even in these situations. The Polyurethane surface, on the other hand, is highly adherent to the soft tissues of the breast making rotation a rare event. In addition, Polyurethane has a role to play in cases of recurrent capsular contracture because of its recognised low contracture rate.

For those concerned about BIA-ALCL, round smooth implants may be the preferred choice. In many situations these may be a very reasonable and appropriate choice where the anatomy is favourable. However, round smooth implants are associated with higher complication and re-operation rates. Both inferior and lateral malpositions are more common as is capsular contracture with the use of smooth surfaces which lack grip and positional stability—this too needs to be discussed with patients.

5.4 Implant Gel/Fill

There is a wide variety of gel fill available amongst different implants. The gel type and characteristics are properties that can be selected in order to confer certain advantages in order to solve particular situations. The advent of form stability as part of the fifth generation devices has led to devices containing more highly cross-linked silicone rendering them more robust and with the ability to maintain their shape better. The form stable or 'gummy bear' gel is also seen as safer in terms of rupture as there is much less fluidity to the gel on breaching of the shell. In general, round implants contain softer gels whilst anatomical implants contain stiffer gels. The latter is true because in order to maintain their shape, anatomical implants have to have a more form stable gel. It is also an important property of anatomical implants—the ability to impart their form on the soft tissues of the breast. A softer gel is more easily compressed by the existing breast tissue whilst a stiffer gel has the opposite effect by imposing its shape on the breast. This form stability combined with the low projection point and volume distribution allows anatomical implants to expand lower poles—either lax or tight and to produce an upward shifting of the nipple-areola complex. The trade-off for the benefits of this increased form stability is a firmer touch.

The latest innovation on gel type is the advent of the B-lite implant; In these implants the silicone gel is bound to air filled borosilicate microspheres rendering the combination approximately 30% lighter than standard silicone gel. The weight reduction is highly appealing to many and especially in secondary cases where the soft tissues are often thin, lax, and lacking in skin thickness and elasticity. The idea of weight reduction in this group is highly desirable. B-lite implants are also the most form stable of all gel types—a property that can be of exploited in trying to solve rippling in thin patients devoid of fat where increased tissue cover is not possible.

The scheme summarises the algorithmic approach to problem solving.

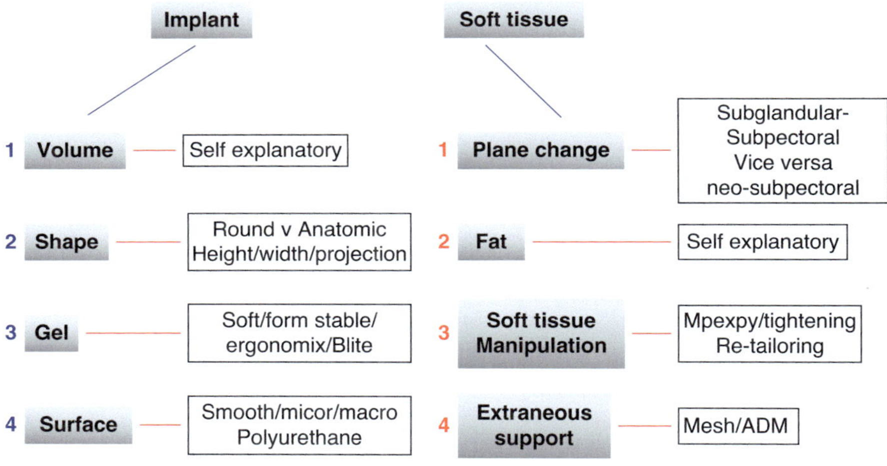

We have devised an abbreviation system based on the above classification, where **I** stands for implant elements and **S** is for soft tissue elements—Each subcategory is allocated a number from 1–4. Therefore, in a case where there has been an exchange of implants from round, smooth to anatomical, textured of the same volume with a plane change from subglandular to subpectoral, the treatment strategy can be summarised as follows: **I (2,4) S (1)**.

The following are two case examples illustrating the use and principles of the IS system (Fig. 1/Case 1 and Fig. 2/Case 2).

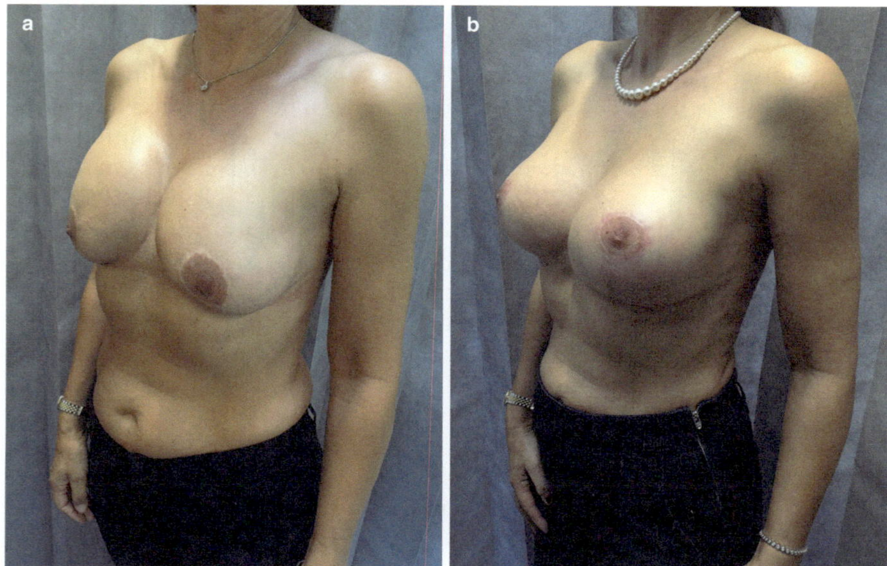

Fig. 1 (**a, b**) Case 1. (**a**) Pre-op. Previous augmentation mastopexy. round smooth implant 150 cc, submuscular unhappy with outcome. Poor volume distribution, too full in upper pole, under filled lower pole. (**b**) Post op. She underwent volume change, shape change, surface change and a redo mastopexy. Using the IS (Implant–Soft tissue) system. I (1) volume change—from 150 to 175 cc, (2) Shape change—from round to anatomical, (4) Surface change—from smooth to Polyurethane (prevent rotation). S (3) revision mastopexy only or to summarise I (1, 2, 4), S (3)

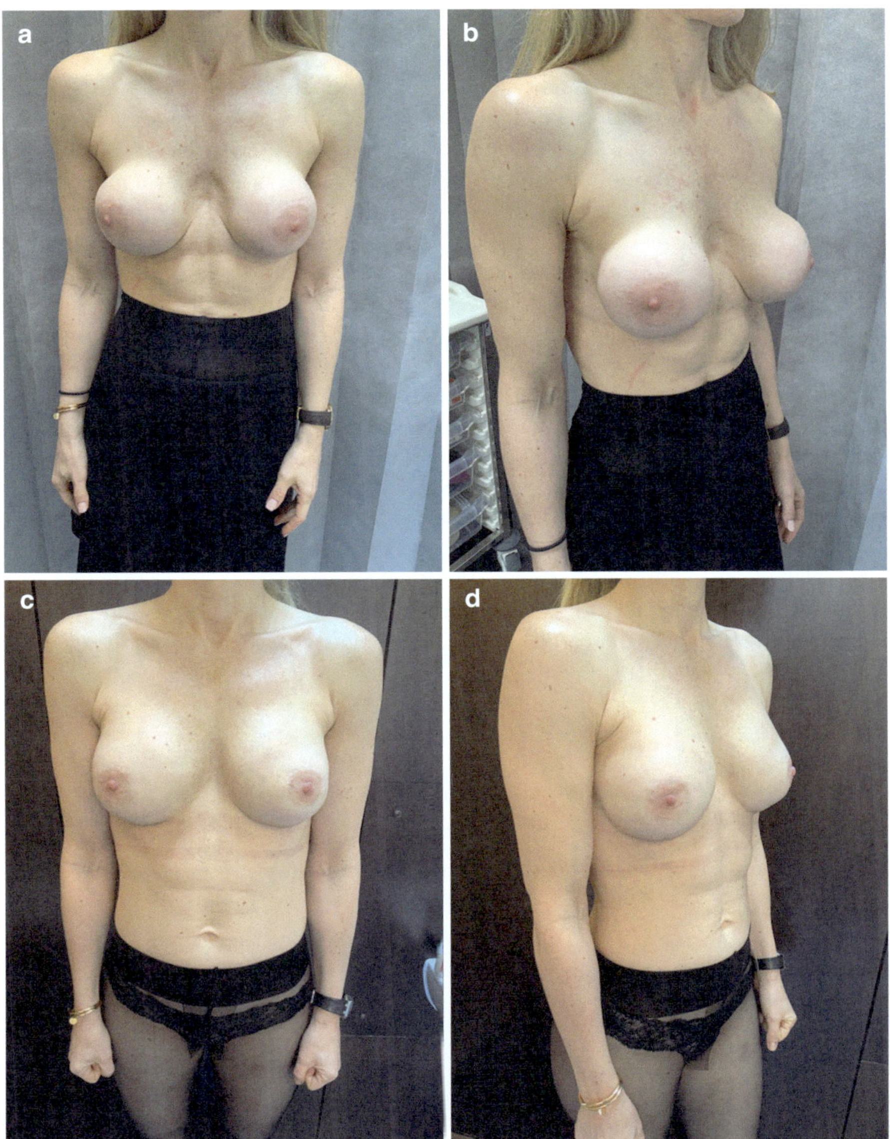

Fig. 2 (a–d) Case 2. Previous augmentation, very unhappy with result, visible, fake looking round textured implants 325 cc, subglandular, rippling, wide cleavage. The plan for surgery was to use a more cohesive gel implant to solve rippling, anatomical shape for a more natural look, polyure-thane coated to avoid rotation, to change the plane from subglandular to subpectoral and add fat transfer to the. cleavage gap. The selected implant was an anatomical B-lite Polyurethane coated, from 325 to 345 cc. Post op changes in summary using the **IS system**. Implant changes: (1) volume change, (2) shape change, (3) gel change, (4) texture change. Soft tissue changes: (1) subglandular to submuscular, (2) fat transfer. Using the IS system it can be summarised as follows **I** (1, 2, 3, 4), **S** (1, 2)

6   Conclusion

Revisional aesthetic breast surgery can be extremely challenging and present with many difficulties. It requires systematic analysis of the problem identifying both soft tissue deficiencies and implant short comings. By compartmentalising the issues, what appear to be highly complex problems can be broken down into simpler ones. Ultimately changes to the soft tissues or the implant or, more commonly, both will help resolve many difficulties. Our simple classification system is a way of not only summarising surgical planning and execution, but also ensuring a systematic way of considering all areas of improvement both in terms of the implant and the soft tissues. It is a means of distilling a complex problem into identifiable and changeable elements.

We firmly believe that the best outcomes in breast augmentation can only be achieved through standardised pre-operative planning of the surgical procedure, a complete knowledge of the available devices, the application of an impeccable surgical technique, and appropriately scheduled follow-up.

The pre-operative planning should reflect a balance between the patient's tissue characteristics and the patient's wishes. The best advice to the patient is that the 'sensible' choice is generally the best one; it respects anatomy and soft tissue boundaries enhancing rather than distorting the breast. Inevitably the best time to get things right is the first time, surgery thereafter only becomes more complicated.

References

1. https://www.fda.gov/medical-devices/breast-implants/update-safety-silicone-gel-filled-breast-implants-2011-executive-summary
2. Wang C, Luan J, Panayi AC, Orgill DP, Xin M. Complications in breast augmentation with textured versus smooth breast implants: a systematic review protocol. BMJ Open. 2018;8(4):e020671. https://doi.org/10.1136/bmjopen-2017-020671. PMID: 29643164; PMCID: PMC5898288.
3. Mallucci PL. 10-year experience using inspira implants: a review with personal anecdote. Plast Reconstr Surg. 2019;144(1S):37S–42S. https://doi.org/10.1097/PRS.0000000000005948. PMID: 31246759.
4. Brown MH, Somogyi RB, Aggarwal S. Secondary breast augmentation. Plast Reconstr Surg. 2016;138(1):119e–35e. https://doi.org/10.1097/PRS.0000000000002280. PMID: 27348674.
5. Calobrace MB, Stevens WG, Capizzi PJ, Cohen R, Godinez T, Beckstrand M. Risk factor analysis for capsular contracture: a 10-year Sientra study using round, smooth, and textured implants for breast augmentation. Plast Reconstr Surg. 2018;141(4S):20S–8S. https://doi.org/10.1097/PRS.0000000000004351. PMID: 29595715.
6. Mallucci P, Branford OA. Design for natural breast augmentation: the ICE principle. Plast Reconstr Surg. 2016;137(6):1728–37. https://doi.org/10.1097/PRS.0000000000002230. PMID: 27219229.
7. Hedén P. Breast augmentation with anatomic, high-cohesiveness silicone gel implants (European experience). In: Spear SL, editor. Surgery of the breast: principles and art. 3rd ed. Philadelphia: Wolters Kluwer/Lippincott Williams & Wilkins; 2011. p. 1322–45.
8. Tebbetts JB, Adams WP. Five critical decisions in breast augmentation using five measurements in 5 minutes: the high five decision support process. Plast Reconstr Surg. 2005;116(7):2005–16. PMID: 16327616.

9. Martin del Yerro JL, Vegas MR, Sanz I. Moreno E, Fernandez V, Puga S, Vecino MG, Biggs TM. Breast augmentation with anatomic implants: a method based on the breast implantation base. Aesthet Plast Surg. 2014;38(2):329–37. https://doi.org/10.1007/s00266-013-0190-5. Epub 2013 Sep 4. PMID: 24002490.

10. Mallucci P, Branford OA. Concepts in aesthetic breast dimensions: analysis of the ideal breast. J Plast Reconstr Aesthet Surg. 2012;65(1):8–16. https://doi.org/10.1016/j.bjps.2011.08.006. Epub 2011 Aug 24. PMID: 21868295.

11. Mallucci P, Branford OA. Population analysis of the perfect breast: a morphometric analysis. Plast Reconstr Surg. 2014;134(3):436–47. https://doi.org/10.1097/PRS.0000000000000485. PMID: 25158703.

12. Adams WP Jr, Culbertson EJ, Deva AK, Magnusson MR, Layt C, Jewell ML, Mallucci P, Hedén P. Macrotextured breast implants with defined steps to minimize bacterial contamination around the device: experience in 42,000 implants. Plast Reconstr Surg. 2017;140(3):427–31. https://doi.org/10.1097/PRS.0000000000003575. PMID: 28841597.

13. Nava MB, Rancati A, Angrigiani C, Catanuto G, Rocco N. How to prevent complications in breast augmentation. Gland Surg. 2017;6(2):210–7. https://doi.org/10.21037/gs.2017.04.02. PMID: 28497025; PMCID: PMC5409896.

14. Maxwell GP, Van Natta BW, Bengtson BP. Murphy DK. Ten-year results from the Natrelle 410 anatomical form-stable silicone breast implant core study. Aesthet Surg J. 2015;35(2):145–55. https://doi.org/10.1093/asj/sju084. Erratum in: Aesthet Surg J. 2015 Nov;35(8):1044. PMID: 25717116; PMCID: PMC4399443.

15. Spear SL, Murphy DK, Allergan Silicone Breast Implant U.S. Core Clinical Study Group. Natrelle round silicone breast implants: core study results at 10 years. Plast Reconstr Surg. 2014;133(6):1354–61. https://doi.org/10.1097/PRS.0000000000000021. PMID: 24867717; PMCID: PMC4819531.

16. Hammond DC, Canady JW, Love TR, Wixtrom RN, Caplin DA. Mentor contour profile gel implants: clinical outcomes at 10 years. Plast Reconstr Surg. 2017;140(6):1142–50. https://doi.org/10.1097/PRS.0000000000003846. PMID: 29176413.

17. Cunningham B, McCue J. Safety and effectiveness of Mentor's MemoryGel implants at 6 years. Aesthetic Plast Surg. 2009;33(3):440–4. https://doi.org/10.1007/s00266-009-9364-6. Epub 2009 May 13. Erratum in: Aesthetic Plast Surg. 2009 May;33(3):439. PMID: 19437068.

18. Maxwell GP, Birchenough SA, Gabriel A. Efficacy of neopectoral pocket in revisionary breast surgery. Aesthet Surg J. 2009;29(5):379–85. https://doi.org/10.1016/j.asj.2009.08.012. PMID: 19825466.

Capsular Contracture

Nick Lahar and William P. Adams Jr

1　Introduction/Background

Since the development of the breast implant in 1962, capsular contracture has been the #1 complication of aesthetic and reconstructive breast surgery [1]. It is also the most common causes of re-operation following implantation.

In addition to operative complications of capsular contracture, there is an economic impact as well. Approximately 1.5 million breast augmentation are done each year outside the US and 300,000 in the US with contracture rate overall between 7 and 15%, resulting in a **staggering 180,000** women affected by capsular contracture each year globally.

There have been numerous theories and treatment strategies for the management of capsular contracture although the subclinical infection etiology has come to the forefront of the science. Other theories include hypertrophic scar hypothesis, activated myofibroblasts, silicone gel bleed, hematoma, or infection related inflammation. Since 1981 [2], Burkhardt demonstrated a connection of sub-acute periprosthetic infection to capsular contracture. In a follow-up prospective study by the same author using randomized clinical split breast design [3], prophylactic treatment of the implants with antibiotic solution demonstrated an 85% reduction in capsular contracture as compared to the opposite untreated side. Although the Burkhardt

N. Lahar
Plastic Surgeon, Beverly Hills, CA, USA

W. P. Adams Jr (✉)
Dallas, TX, USA

Plastic Surgery UT Southwestern Medical Center Dallas, TX, USA
e-mail: wpajrmd@dr-adams.com

© Springer Nature Switzerland AG 2022
R. de Vita (ed.), *Aesthetic Breast Augmentation Revision Surgery*,
https://doi.org/10.1007/978-3-030-86793-5_2

study first implicated Staph epidermidis, further studies have implicated multiple bacterial types in the formation of capsular contracture. Staph epidermidis is certainly the most mentioned species, but *P. acnes*, *E. coli,* and other bacteria have been cultured from capsular contracture pockets [4, 5]. Histologic examination of capsules and the implants were initially inconsistent, demonstrating no bacteria with "typical" swabs of the implant pocket. Examinations of the capsules using electron microscopy revealed little evidence of bacteria in the capsules, perhaps from sampling error and tenacious biofilms [6]. Some of these studies may have slowed our understanding of bacteria inoculation as a significant etiology for capsular contracture. There was mounting evidence in other medical subspecialties that bacterial biofilm formation was a ubiquitous phenomenon affecting various medical devices [7], urinary catheters [8], central lines, and orthopedic implants. Biofilms are ubiquitous and these studies helped clarify an etiology for capsular contracture [9]. Increasingly sophisticated studies helped our understanding of bacteria/ biofilm as the key cause:effect factor in capsular contracture [10, 11]. Through all of these investigations the process of capsular contracture has been elucidated: inoculation of the implant and implant pocket with a biologically significant mass of bacteria, attachment and accumulation of the bacteria on implant surfaces, formation of the antibiotic resistant protective biofilm, and subsequent low grade inflammatory response by the local host, manifests as pathologic and progressive capsular contracture. Additionally, our understanding of capsular contracture and its relation to the microbiome has helped us better understand what is still a currently hotly investigated topic, Breast Implant Associated-Anaplastic Large Cell Lymphoma (BIA-ALCL).

As capsular contracture remains the most common complication, surgeons see patients for revision of this malady very often and it is the #1 most common reason for revision breast augmentation. Although this chapter will concentrate on the surgical treatment of contracture, surgeons should keep in mind that **the best defense of contracture is a good offense**. We will start with prevention as these concepts are critical to the management of existing capsular contracture.

2 Key Concepts in Capsular Contracture Prevention/ Prophylaxis

An ounce of prevention is worth a pound of cure.
  Benjamin Franklin

The concept that **Bacteria are Bad and More Bacteria are Worse** is a simple, yet powerful dictum. Bacteria produce the chronic inflammation that result in the fibrotic response that we call capsular contracture. We now know that depending on the specific type of bacteria, there can be other host responses including a transformative response resulting in BIA-ALCL. Prevention of bacterial contamination will reduce these divergent consequences prior to their development.

2.1 The Science of Capsular Contracture: Subclinical Infection

The connection between capsular contracture and bacterial contamination of the implant was first described in the 1980s. Because of their suspicions of subclinical Staphylococcus epidermidis infection as a potential cause of capsular contracture, Shah et al. [12] demonstrated significant contracture in rabbit implant pockets inoculated with the bacteria. During the same time, Burkhardt et al. [3] demonstrated a 50% reduction in capsular contracture with the introduction of antibiotic irrigation into the breast pocket prior to the insertion of implants using intrapatient controls. A retrospective review by Netscher et al. [13] of 389 implants removed for reasons other than overt infection correlated positive staphylococcus with the development of significant III/IV capsular contractures. Their study refers to a review of the formation of biofilms in other medical specialties [14] and references the relative difficulty of obtaining a "standard culture" of breast implant pockets due to the protective biofilm layer that entraps offending pathogens. A stronger argument was made by Pajkos et al. (2003) in a prospective clinical trial examining the relationship of biofilm associated bacterial colonization and capsular contracture in patients having implant explantation. Routine culture swabs of the breast pockets were negative in all examined pockets. Using a more thorough ultrasonification of the capsules, 17/19 implants with Baker III/IV capsular contracture were positive for coag-negative Staph whereas only 1/8 Baker I/II capsules were culture positive. The group used electron microscopy to demonstrate bacterial species interspersed within extensive biofilm. These data help to clarify bacterial inoculation as a major, if not the most important, cause of capsular contracture. No other etiology has come close to explaining capsular contracture development although other inflammatory factors may play a potentiating role [15].

Further studies of the bacteria-implant-capsule interaction have brought about new understandings of the patient immune response and the effect texturing has upon the clinical response. Texturization of implants was developed as a means for reducing capsular contracture following the introduction of polyurethane-foam covered implants, although this logic has now been disproven. Various studies comparing smooth and textured implants showed either modest reduction of capsular contracture [16] or no improvement [17, 18]. Proponents of texturing argue the texturing allows improved integration of the host tissues into the textured surface of the implant. Other studies suggest there is improved fibroblast adhesion, and blood supply to the immediate area [19–21]. To investigate the effect texturing had upon biofilm development, Jacombs et al. [22] used the well-establish porcine model to evaluate a total of 121 smooth or textured implants, with 66 implants inoculated with Staphylococcus epidermidis. In this study, there was no difference in the rates of capsular contracture for inoculated smooth vs. textured implants with about 80% capsular contracture rate in these groups. However, at 2, 6, and 24 h, the textured implants demonstrated a 11-,43-, and 72-fold higher bacterial load on the surface compared to smooth implants. The contracted implants had a 250-fold higher number of bacteria in the capsules, whether from smooth or textured implants. Furthermore, clinical studies have demonstrated less capsular contracture in smooth vs. textured implants [23, 24]. All of these studies underscore the issue that many surgeons have followed for years mistakenly believing textured implants cause less capsular contracture. This reduction is not supported by data consistently and the increase surface area of the texture increases the amount of bacteria which may cause an increased risk for capsular contracture and also other bacterially mediated processes, specifically BIA-ALCL [24].

2.2   An Ounce of Prevention: Minimizing the Development of Capsular Contracture

With the science of capsular contracture firmly implicating subclinical infection as the major cause, groups began to investigate optimal means of reducing bioburden. An animal study by Tamboto, et al. inoculating porcine mammary pockets with Staph epidermidis demonstrated capsular contracture with bacterial inoculation, consistent with the studies mentioned above. However, the study also suggested that that below a certain bacterial threshold, capsular contracture may not occur [11]. There is merit in reducing to the best of our ability the bacterial burden at the time of surgery. A easy means for surgeons to do this would be minimizing bacterial load in the breast pocket with antimicrobial breast pocket irrigation that would bring the critical bacterial threshold to a low enough point to minimize the infectious contribution to capsular contracture. Given the polymicrobial nature of device associated infection (capsular contracture, BIA-ALCL, seroma etc). The ideal breast irrigant would maximally reduce bacterial numbers (broad spectrum), minimally cytotoxic, have relatively available ingredients, be easy to create. While surgeons were recognizing the role of bacterial contamination and capsular contracture, there was no standardization in the practice of breast pocket preparation that was clinically proven to reduce bacterial numbers and reduce capsular contracture. Adams et al [25] sought to optimize and standardize breast pocket irrigation. Their concern was that surgeons were conscious of the importance of antibiotic irrigation (at least for the reduction of acute infection) but there was no gold standard nor standardization of technique. They evaluated various antibiotic combinations in vitro that would neutralize the most common bacterial species cultured from implants and implicated in capsular contracture (P. acnes, S. epidermidis, E. coli) as well as species implicated in more acute infections (S. aureus, P. aeruginosa) [5]. The result was a recommendation of either Betadine Triple (BT) (50 ml of povidone-iodine, 1 g of cefazolin, and 80 mg of gentamicin in 500 mL) or 50% Betadine [25] and then a year later after betadine was label-restricted in the FDA saline implant PMA hearings, a non-betadine triple antibiotic (NB-TAB) (50,000 U Bacitracin, 1 g cefazolin, 80 mg gentamicin, 500 cc NS) [26]. The same irrigations BT, 50% betadine, and NB-TAB were then evaluated clinically in a 6-year prospective study that examined the rate of capsular contracture in breast augmentation, reconstruction, and augmentation mastopexy. Capsular contraction rates were 1.8% (5x lower), 9.5% (9x lower), and 0%, significantly below previous series [27–29]. A 20-year follow-up study by the same group has demonstrated further decreases in capsular contracture of 0.57%.

Deva, Adams and Vickery and [30] suammarized recommendations that address the clinical data regarding breast implants and minimization of bacterial load. These recommendations are summarized in a "14 point plan" that aim to ultimately minimize and prevent capsular contracture formation. Each point uses data to support its inclusion on the list. The points are as follows:

1. Use intravenous antibiotic prophylaxis at the time of anesthetic induction.
2. Avoid periareolar incisions; these have been shown in both laboratory and clinical studies to lead to a higher rate of contracture as the pocket dissection is contaminated directly by bacteria within the breast tissue.
3. Use nipple shields to prevent spillage of bacteria into the pocket.
4. Perform careful atraumatic dissection to minimize devascularized tissue.
5. Perform careful hemostasis.
6. Avoid dissection into the breast parenchyma. The use of a dual plane, subfascial pocket has anatomic advantages.
7. Perform pocket irrigation with triple antibiotic solution or betadine.
8. Minimize skin-implant contamination.
9. Use new instruments and drapes, and change surgical gloves prior to handling the implant.
10. Minimize the time of implant opening.
11. Minimize repositioning and replacement of the implant.
12. Use a layered closure.
13. Avoid using a drainage tube, which can be a potential site of entry for bacteria.
14. Use antibiotic prophylaxis to cover subsequent procedures that breach skin or mucosa.

These points can be applied easily to a well-defined surgical process [31] in both primary and revisionary breast surgery without significant additional time commitment. All of these interventions can be performed with supplies readily available in most any surgical center.

We recommend to our patients antibiotic prophylaxis to cover subsequent procedures that breach skin/mucosa such as dental procedures. Ellenbogen suggested a causal relation between dental prophylaxis and rapid breast encapsulation within weeks of the surgical procedure based on personal experience [32]. Within the dental and orthopedic literature, there is mixed clinical data with regard to antibiotic prophylaxis for patients at risk for bacterial endocarditis or seeding of orthopedic implants [33]. The general consensus in these papers recommend discussion of risk versus benefit with patients. Given the relative infrequency of these procedures, the reduction of transient bacteremia would potentially impart some protective measures.

The 14 Point Plan's effectiveness was examined using pooled data from eight plastic surgeons performing breast augmentation with macrotextured implants from multiple areas globally using the above described technique. The study reported a low capsular contracture rates of 2.2% in 42,035 macrotexture implantations over a mean follow-up of 10 years. Additionally, the expected # of BIA-ALCL cases was 15 and the actual # of BIA-ALCL cases in the study was zero. The study supports the role of surgical technique in risk reduction of BIA-ALCL [34].

3 Management of Capsular Contracture

Although the rates of capsular contracture have decreased significantly over the years with rates reported as low as 1% [34] with the interventions mentioned above, plastic surgeons will be faced with these patients despite best practices. Capsular contracture has been typically graded on the Baker scale with Baker Grades I and II typically being managed conservatively and Baker III and IV grades managed surgically.

Non-surgical means of treating capsular contracture have been employed to minimize progression. The most commonly mentioned medications are the leukotriene inhibitors such as zafirlukast (Accolate; AstraZeneca, London, United Kingdom) and montelukast (Singulair; Merck, Kenilworth, N.J.). In Scuderi's preliminary report, 20 women were examined and the study's conclusion was that zafirlukast may reduce pain and breast capsule distortion for patients with long-standing contracture. One conclusion was that this drug could potentially be offered to patients who either are not surgical candidates or do not wish to undergo surgery [35]. In a follow-up long-term study, the group demonstrated improvement in breast capsule distortion while the drug was being taken but increased contracture once the drug was no longer taken. More concerning, however, is that the safety profile of the drug is not benign. There is a risk of hepatotoxicity and other side effects. The drug (used off-label) also simply treats the symptoms of the capsular contracture but as demonstrated above, does not address the root cause for the problem. While they may have a role in patients unwilling or unable to undergo surgery, leukotriene inhibitors are not a mainstay of treatment for capsular contracture.

Surgery is the primary modality for treatment of Baker III and IV type capsular contracture. Our preferred surgical algorithm is summarized in Fig. 1.

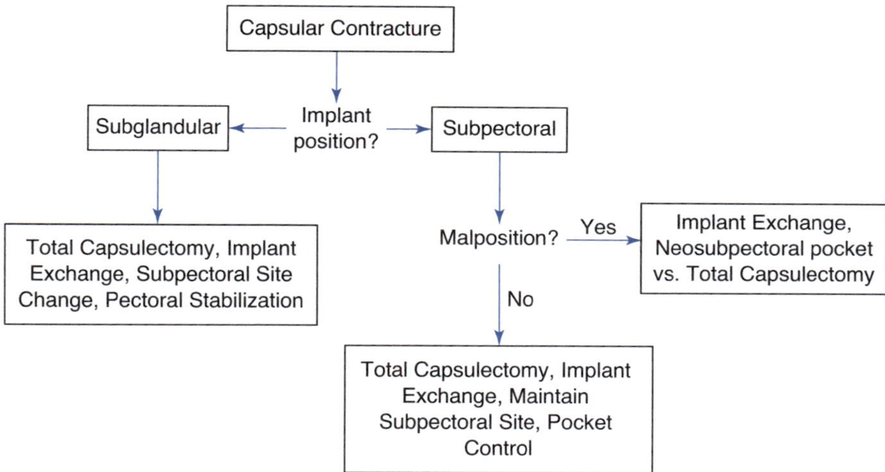

Fig. 1 This simple algorithm for capsular contracture stratifies treatment based on some glandular vs. subpectoral position. The gold standard is total, precise capsulectomy, implant exchange in a subpectoral pocket. If malposition is also present a Neo subpectoral pocket is the preferred technique

Historically, there is a generalized dogma for capsular contracture: capsulectomy, site change, and implant exchange; however, there are multiple factors that should be assessed when evaluating a surgical candidate. These include implant site, presence of malposition, tissue quality, and implant type. Management should be geared toward the patient's personal clinical scenario. We present decision points in management. With regard to the data in breast surgery, we find much of it to be, while good intentioned, non-specific in surgical technique and not transferrable. Vastly varying recurring contracture rates can be found in the literature. There are some studies that do offer insights into management of capsular contracture and we include some here to help us in our decision-making.

4   Precise Total Capsulectomy Versus Partial Capsulectomy Versus Capsulotomy

Precise total capsulectomy involves the complete removal of the contracted capsule while partial capsulotomy refers to a subtotal excision, usually the anterior leaf of the capsule. Capsulotomy refers to the divsion of the capsule with the goal to break the continuity of fibrous scar but leaving the majority of the capsule within the pocket.

Much of the data gathering, surgical management, and follow-up related to capsulotomy versus capsulectomy is heterogeneous and the recurrence rates are widely divergent with a range of 0–53% [36–38]. In the most definitive study comparing anterior versus total capsulectomy, Collis and Sharpe [36, 39] demonstrated recurrent capsular contracture in 46% of patients treated with only anterior capsulectomy versus 11% in the total capsulectomy group. Capsules demonstrating contracture have repeatedly demonstrated significant levels of biofilm and associated bacteria when processed appropriately [10] and to leave them adjacent to a new implant and pocket sets up an environment for contracture recurrence. Since we know that bacteria are the most significant contributor to capsular contracture, why would we leave an affected capsule? Additionally, there is also data to suggest that a site change using a neosubpectoral pocket, excluding the old capsular contracture pocket from the new implant space, does not predispose to recurrent capsular contracture [40].

Essentially, if performed appropriately, the new implant interface does not encounter the previous contaminated pocket, but is merely adjacent to it. Maintaining this isolation of the new implant from the old pocket is key to reducing recurrence.

We recommend that precise total capsulectomy be performed whenever possible. We find that it is rare for a precise total capsulectomy to be difficult to perform. If the posterior leaf is adherent to the chest wall, hydrodissection can facilitate lift of the capsule safely.

5   Site Change Vs. No Site Change

The surgeon can choose to maintain the location of the implant or perform a site change. The site of the implant can be divided into the following: subpectoral, subglandular, or neosubpectoral. There are multiple studies that find a low capsular contracture recurrence rate with site change [40–43]. Additionally, the best data is consistent with placement of new implants under the muscle [44, 45].

For a subglandular implant with associated capsular contracture, we recommend precise total capsulectomy, site change implant, or removal. If an implant is still desired, we strongly recommend replacement of the old implant with a new implant in order to not re-introduce a high bacterial load contaminated implant into the pocket. As stressed above, implant biofilms are tenacious and difficult to eradicate. A site change is performed with placement of the new implant under the pectoralis muscle. Since the subglandular space has been undermined, there is risk of window shading of the pectoralis superiorly, as in an aggressive dual plane breast augmentation. The lower edge of the pectoralis muscle can be controlled with a sheet of acellular dermal matrix, or natural scaffold (typically P4HB) mesh, to recreate the normal virgin anatomy as much as possible [46–48]. We typically use a drain to minimize seroma formation under the raw subglandular space, as well. We have a low threshold for staging any secondary mastopexy procedures in these cases given the violation of the intercostal perforators and extent of dissection.

For a submuscular implant with associated capsular contracture, we also recommend precise total capsulectomy and implant exchange or removal in the subpectoral space. If an implant is still desired, we strongly recommend replacement of the old implant with a new implant in order to not re-introduce a contaminated implant into the pocket. We maintain the subpectoral position of the implant and do not perform a site change in this case. We will perform a dual plane adjustment as necessary for the outcome. We typically use a drain to minimize seroma formation given the significant raw subpectoral space, as well.

If there is concern that risk of elevation of the posterior leaf of the capsule will be difficult and the capsule is thick, a neosubpectoral pocket can be used to create a new pocket for the new implant. The neosubpectoral pocket can also be useful in cases of malposition. A new dissection outside of the malpositioned pocket can be carefully crafted to fit a new implant in the exact position desired. This technique offers a significant degree of control of the pocket size. The capsule space should be obliterated with electrocautery and stitches through the anterior and posterior leaves to minimize seroma formation. Conceptually, it is important to completely exclude the contaminated pocket by dissecting between the posterior pectoralis and the anterior capsule and to minimize holes/tears that may introduce bacteria secondarily from the old pocket into the new pocket.

Special mention should be made of ADM and reports of reduced capsular contracture rates [46, 49]. While ADM offers a form of pocket control and possible contour improvement if necessary, it has been in our experience that it does not always prevent the formation of capsular contracture in revisionary surgeries we have encountered. Currently, there is some evolving data on the utility of P4HB in the prevention of recurrent capsular contracture and time will tell on its true efficacy. Cost with these adjuncts [50]. Cost is also a factor for these adjuncts.

6 Conclusion

Capsular contracture has been the #1 risk of breast augmentation surgery since the breast implants became avaible in 1963. Advances in our understanding of the etiology for capsular contracture and an evidence-based, surgical process have dropped the rates of capsular contracture by all measures to less than 1%. Patient outcomes have improved. However, because of the heterogeneity of surgical practice and patient factors, capsular contracture is still the most common cause of re-operative breast surgery. By optimizing revisional surgery, a second chance is offered to "get it right." The same techniques that minimize capsular contracture also reduce other device associated infection issues including breast implant associated ALCL.

References

1. Handel N, Cordray T, Gutierrez J, Jensen JA. A long-term study of outcomes, complications, and patient satisfaction with breast implants. Plast Reconstr Surg. 2006;117(3):757–67; discussion 768–772.
2. Burkhardt BR, Fried M, Schnur PL, Tofield JJ. Capsules, infection, and intraluminal antibiotics. Plast Reconstr Surg. 1981;68(1):43–9.
3. Burkhardt BR, Dempsey PD, Schnur PL, Tofield JJ. Capsular contracture: a prospective study of the effect of local antibacterial agents. Plast Reconstr Surg. 1986;77(6):919–32.
4. Dobke MK, Svahn JK, Vastine VL, Landon BN, Stein PC, Parsons CL. Characterization of microbial presence at the surface of silicone mammary implants. Ann Plast Surg. 1995;34(6):563–9; discussion 570–561.
5. Ahn CY, Ko CY, Wagar EA, Wong RS, Shaw WW. Microbial evaluation: 139 implants removed from symptomatic patients. Plast Reconstr Surg. 1996;98(7):1225–9.
6. Rudolph R, Woodward M. Absence of visible bacteria in capsules around silicone breast implants. Plast Reconstr Surg. 1983;72(1):32–7.
7. Bryers JD. Medical biofilms. Biotechnol Bioeng. 2008;100(1):1–18.
8. Rogers J, Norkett DI, Bracegirdle P, et al. Examination of biofilm formation and risk of infection associated with the use of urinary catheters with leg bags. J Hosp Infect. 1996;32(2):105–15.
9. Costerton JW, Montanaro L, Arciola CR. Biofilm in implant infections: its production and regulation. Int J Artif Organs. 2005;28(11):1062–8.
10. Pajkos A, Deva AK, Vickery K, Cope C, Chang L, Cossart YE. Detection of subclinical infection in significant breast implant capsules. Plast Reconstr Surg. 2003;111(5):1605–11.
11. Tamboto H, Vickery K, Deva AK. Subclinical (biofilm) infection causes capsular contracture in a porcine model following augmentation mammaplasty. Plast Reconstr Surg. 2010;126(3):835–42.
12. Shah Z, Lehman JA Jr, Tan J. Does infection play a role in breast capsular contracture? Plast Reconstr Surg. 1981;68(1):34–42.
13. Netscher DT, Weizer G, Wigoda P, Walker LE, Thornby J, Bowen D. Clinical relevance of positive breast periprosthetic cultures without overt infection. Plast Reconstr Surg. 1995;96(5):1125–9.
14. van Loosdrecht MC, Lyklema J, Norde W, Zehnder AJ. Influence of interfaces on microbial activity. Microbiol Rev. 1990;54(1):75–87.

15. Adams WP Jr. Capsular contracture: what is it? What causes it? How can it be prevented and managed? Clin Plast Surg. 2009;36(1):119–26, vii.
16. Burkhardt BR, Eades E. The effect of biocell texturing and povidone-iodine irrigation on capsular contracture around saline-inflatable breast implants. Plast Reconstr Surg. 1995;96(6):1317–25.
17. Fagrell D, Berggren A, Tarpila E. Capsular contracture around saline-filled fine textured and smooth mammary implants: a prospective 7.5-year follow-up. Plast Reconstr Surg. 2001;108(7):2108–12; discussion 2113.
18. Tarpila E, Ghassemifar R, Fagrell D, Berggren A. Capsular contracture with textured versus smooth saline-filled implants for breast augmentation: a prospective clinical study. Plast Reconstr Surg. 1997;99(7):1934–9.
19. Xu LC, Siedlecki CA. Submicron-textured biomaterial surface reduces staphylococcal bacterial adhesion and biofilm formation. Acta Biomater. 2012;8(1):72–81.
20. Clubb FJ Jr, Clapper DL, Deferrari DA, et al. Surface texturing and coating of biomaterial implants: effects on tissue integration and fibrosis. ASAIO J. 1999;45(4):281–7.
21. Dalby MJ, Yarwood SJ, Riehle MO, Johnstone HJ, Affrossman S, Curtis AS. Increasing fibroblast response to materials using nanotopography: morphological and genetic measurements of cell response to 13-nm-high polymer demixed islands. Exp Cell Res. 2002;276(1):1–9.
22. Jacombs A, Tahir S, Hu H, et al. In vitro and in vivo investigation of the influence of implant surface on the formation of bacterial biofilm in mammary implants. Plast Reconstruct Surg. 2014;133(4):471e–80e.
23. Stoff-Khalili MA, Scholze R, Morgan WR, Metcalf JD. Subfascial periareolar augmentation mammaplasty. Plast Reconstr Surg. 2004;114(5):1280–8; discussion 1289–1291.
24. Lahar N, Adams Jr. WP. Optimizing breast pocket irrigation—21 year follow-up. Paper presented at: annual meeting of the American Society of Aesthetic Plastic Surgery 2018. New York, NY.
25. Adams WP Jr, Conner WC, Barton FE Jr, Rohrich RJ. Optimizing breast pocket irrigation: an in vitro study and clinical implications. Plast Reconstr Surg. 2000;105(1):334–8; discussion 339–343.
26. Adams WP Jr, Conner WC, Barton FE Jr, Rohrich RJ. Optimizing breast-pocket irrigation: the post-betadine era. Plast Reconstr Surg. 2001;107(6):1596–601.
27. Adams WP Jr, Rios JL, Smith SJ. Enhancing patient outcomes in aesthetic and reconstructive breast surgery using triple antibiotic breast irrigation: six-year prospective clinical study. Plast Reconstr Surg. 2006;117(1):30–6.
28. Blount AL, Martin MD, Lineberry KD, Kettaneh N, Alfonso DR. Capsular contracture rate in a low-risk population after primary augmentation mammaplasty. Aesthet Surg J. 2013;33(4):516–21.
29. Giordano S, Peltoniemi H, Lilius P, Salmi A. Povidone-iodine combined with antibiotic topical irrigation to reduce capsular contracture in cosmetic breast augmentation: a comparative study. Aesthet Surg J. 2013;33(5):675–80.
30. Deva AK, Adams WP Jr, Vickery K. The role of bacterial biofilms in device-associated infection. Plast Reconstr Surg. 2013;132(5):1319–28.
31. Tebbetts JB. Achieving a predictable 24-hour return to normal activities after breast augmentation: part II. Patient preparation, refined surgical techniques, and instrumentation. Plast Reconstr Surg. 2002;109(1):293–305; discussion 306–397.
32. Ellenbogen R. Breast implant encapsulation in association with dental work. Plast Reconstr Surg. 1986;78(4):541.
33. Glenny AM, Oliver R, Roberts GJ, Hooper L, Worthington HV. Antibiotics for the prophylaxis of bacterial endocarditis in dentistry. Cochrane Database Syst Rev. 2013;(10):CD003813.
34. Adams W Jr, Culbertson EJ, Deva AK, Magnusson M, Layt C, Jewell M, Mallucci P, Heden P. Macrotextured breast implants with defined steps to minimize bacterial contamination around the device—experience in 42,000 implants. Plast Reconstr Surg. 2017;140(3):427–31.
35. Scuderi N, Mazzocchi M, Fioramonti P, Bistoni G. The effects of zafirlukast on capsular contracture: preliminary report. Aesthet Plast Surg. 2006;30(5):513–20.

36. Costagliola M, Atiyeh BS, Rampillon F. An innovative procedure for the treatment of primary and recurrent capsular contracture (CC) following breast augmentation. Aesthet Surg J. 2013;33(7):1008–17.
37. Abazov VM, Abbott B, Abdesselam A, et al. Search for narrow tt resonances in pp collisions at square root of (s)=1.8 TeV. Phys Rev Lett. 2004;92(22):221801.
38. Hester TR Jr, Ghazi BH, Moyer HR, Nahai FR, Wilton M, Stokes L. Use of dermal matrix to prevent capsular contracture in aesthetic breast surgery. Plast Reconstr Surg. 2012;130(5 Suppl 2):126S–36S.
39. Collis N, Sharpe DT. Recurrence of subglandular breast implant capsular contracture: anterior versus total capsulectomy. Plast Reconstr Surg. 2000;106(4):792–7.
40. Maxwell GP, Birchenough SA, Gabriel A. Efficacy of neopectoral pocket in revisionary breast surgery. Aesthet Surg J. 2009;29(5):379–85.
41. Castello MF, Lazzeri D, Silvestri A, et al. Maximizing the use of precapsular space and the choice of implant type in breast augmentation mammaplasty revisions: review of 49 consecutive procedures and patient satisfaction assessment. Aesthet Plast Surg. 2011;35(5):828–38.
42. Xue H, Lee SY. Correction of capsular contracture by insertion of a breast prosthesis anterior to the original capsule and preservation of the contracted capsule: technique and outcomes. Aesthet Plast Surg. 2011;35(6):1056–60.
43. Lee HK, Jin US, Lee YH. Subpectoral and precapsular implant repositioning technique: correction of capsular contracture and implant malposition. Aesthet Plast Surg. 2011;35(6):1126–32.
44. Schaub TA, Ahmad J, Rohrich RJ. Capsular contracture with breast implants in the cosmetic patient: saline versus silicone—a systematic review of the literature. Plast Reconstr Surg. 2010;126(6):2140–9.
45. Barnsley GP, Sigurdson LJ, Barnsley SE. Textured surface breast implants in the prevention of capsular contracture among breast augmentation patients: a meta-analysis of randomized controlled trials. Plast Reconstr Surg. 2006;117(7):2182–90.
46. Basu CB, Jeffers L. The role of acellular dermal matrices in capsular contracture: a review of the evidence. Plast Reconstr Surg. 2012;130(5 Suppl 2):118S–24S.
47. Maxwell GP, Gabriel A. Acellular dermal matrix in aesthetic revisionary breast surgery. Aesthet Surg J. 2011;31(7 Suppl):65S–76S.
48. Chasan PE. Breast capsulorrhaphy revisited: a simple technique for complex problems. Plast Reconstr Surg. 2005;115(1):296–301; discussion 302–393
49. Maxwell GP, Gabriel A. Use of the acellular dermal matrix in revisionary aesthetic breast surgery. Aesthet Surg J. 2009;29(6):485–93.
50. Sigalove S, Maxwell GP, Sigalove NM, et al. Prepectoral implant-based breast reconstruction: rationale, indications, and preliminary results. Plast Reconstr Surg. 2017;139(2):287–94.

Shape Deformities After Breast Augmentation: Double Bubble, Bottoming Out, and Wrinkling

Phillip Blondeel

1 Introduction: The 3-Step Principle

In 2009 my co-authors and I have published a universal system [1–4] for the approach of all types of aesthetic and reconstructive surgery in order to achieve aesthetically pleasing results. This applies specifically to redo breast augmentation surgery.

The 3-step principle helps surgeons to analyze a problematic breast by understanding the three main anatomical features of a breast and how they interact: the footprint, the conus of the breast, and the skin envelope. The analytical approach that we have described allows the experienced and novice plastic surgeon to break down, understand, and describe the different deformities present in a troubled breast, whatever the cause might be. With a better comprehension of what is wrong with the size and shape of the breast, the same surgical philosophy (the "three-step" principle) can be applied to perform a systematic and step-by-step improvement or reconstruction leading to an aesthetically pleasing and reproducible result. By breaking down the breast into the three structures described below, we can easily analyze the problems present at each of these levels and devise a surgical strategy for correcting the different issues at the three levels and creating an aesthetically pleasing breast.

Today, I will use this 3-step principle for every single case of breast surgery, easy or complex. Specially in those cases where you have the feeling that you cannot put your finger on the problem immediately, this systematic approach will help you to find a solution instantly.

P. Blondeel (✉)
Department of Plastic Surgery, Ghent University Hospital, Ghent, Belgium
e-mail: Phillip.blondeel@ugent.be

© Springer Nature Switzerland AG 2022
R. de Vita (ed.), *Aesthetic Breast Augmentation Revision Surgery*,
https://doi.org/10.1007/978-3-030-86793-5_3

1.1 Breast Footprint

The breast "footprint" is the outline or footprint that the breast makes on the chest wall, analogous to the footprint a tent makes on the ground. The footprint forms the basis or foundation of the overlying three-dimensional structure of the breast (Fig. 1). This footprint may vary individually in height and width. Also, the position of the footprint on the chest wall may vary slightly from one woman to another, but mostly the borders of the footprint are related to well-known anatomical structures on the chest wall.

It is important to understand that the footprint will never change in the same woman either in position or in dimensions after puberty. When the breast becomes larger because of hormonal influences or weight gain, the breast will never grow over the midaxillary line, the inframammary crease, the midline, or up to the clavicle. Gravity may pull on the soft tissues, hereby descending the mammary structures in a caudal direction but no more than a few millimeters to centimeters. Establishing an appropriate footprint is the first step in both aesthetic and reconstructive surgery.

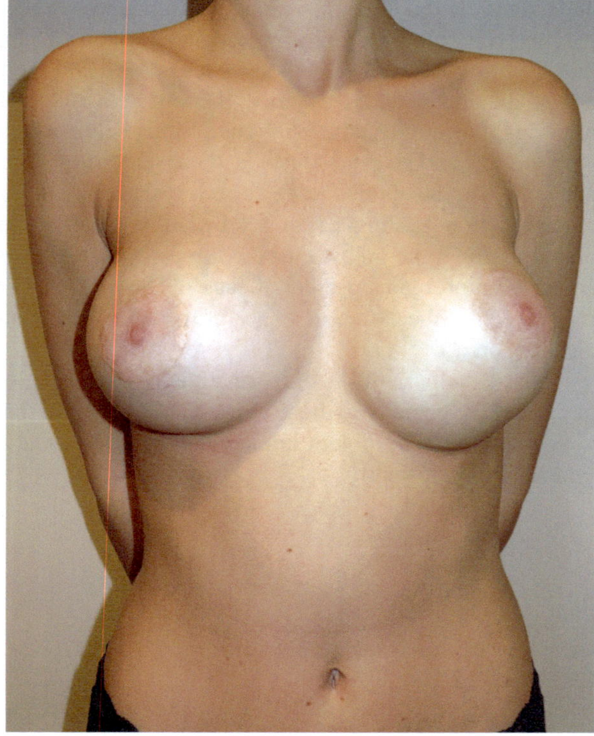

Fig. 1 Example of a distortion of the lower border of the footprint, being the inframammary crease. There is a minimal downward shift of the upper border. All other borders of the footprint are symmetrical with the contralateral side

1.2   Breast Conus

The breast conus refers to the three-dimensional shape, projection, and volume of the tissue (or implant) on top and anterior to the footprint of the breast. This conus has a very specific volume distribution yet is different in each individual woman. An aesthetic breast is inherently asymmetric, with a greater proportion of its volume residing in the lower pole of the breast. Although the breast footprint is relatively similar from one patient to the next. the breast conus differs significantly from patient to patient and with age. This is demonstrated most obviously when looking at breasts with different degrees of hypertrophy or ptosis.

The basis of the conus corresponds or is slightly smaller than the breast footprint. The conus will also need an inferolateral fullness, which defines the lower outer quadrant of the breast, a maximum projection in an anteroposterior direction in its lower part at the level of the nipple-areola complex and some degree of ptosis. The degree of medial fullness and the angle of the conus at its medial border will determine the amount of medial cleavage possible but only in conjunction with the medial position of the breast footprint.

An aesthetic breast is virtually impossible to create without an appropriately established footprint that serves as the foundation for the overlying breast conus. The conus shape and volume may vary from one woman to another and needs to be adjusted and remodeled to achieve final symmetry with the contralateral side.

1.3   The Breast Envelope

The quantity and quality of the skin envelope have a major influence on breast aesthetics (Fig. 3). A skin envelope of appropriate quantity functions like a well-fitting brassiere, holding the parenchymal volume, or conus, in an appropriate position. Both in a vertical and horizontal direction, the exact amount of skin is necessary to create a nice shape. Any redundancy of skin in any direction will lead to awkward breast shapes and to (early) ptosis. Skin shortage or overtightening will lead to flattening of the breast, wound-healing problems, or even necrosis of the underlying autologous tissue.

A skin envelope of appropriate quality has good elasticity and a certain firmness allowing and assisting in appropriate projection of the (parenchymal) tissue. Once the skin envelope has lost a significant degree of elasticity, the skin will stretch and the breast will appear ptotic even if the parenchymal volume and shape are maintained. Irradiation and previous scars both influence the skin envelope, causing it to be tighter and less elastic.

One also has to consider that, at the interface between the envelope and the conus, a variable interaction will take place. In case of autologous tissue, variable amounts of scar will form, depending on the type of surgery and on possible complications such as hematomas and infections. In case of implants, a capsule will form. This capsule will not interact directly with the skin but might displace or deform the conus. The skin envelope will not have sufficient strength to counteract this process and will follow the changes in the capsule.

The final shape of the breast is never determined by the footprint, the conus, or the envelope independently. It is the combined action of these three elements that will result in a pleasing and natural-appearing breast that maintains a stable shape over years.

## 2	Double Bubble

### 2.1	Etiology

A double bubble deformity can be caused by a shortage of skin envelope, a shortage of conus, or by traction of an upward moving origin of the pectoral muscle.

### 2.1.1	Shortage of Skin

The most commonly known pathology is the tubular breast deformity that presents itself with a variable underdevelopment of one or both lower quadrants. This deformity also comes in variable degrees. In mild cases the lack of glandular tissue and lack of skin is minimal and optimal results can be achieved with minimal surgical effort. In others, there may be an important underdevelopment of glandular tissue, followed by insufficient anterior propulsion and insufficient stretch of the skin envelope.

The most important cause of iatrogenic double bubble deformity is every case where an implant, or in rare cases also autologous tissue like lipofilling or an autologous flap, is placed under and below the inframammary crease and where there is insufficient expansion of the skin envelope in a horizontal direction at the level of that inframammary crease. There is insufficient skin in a horizontal direction for the volume of the conus. A shortage of skin can also be caused by excessive removal of skin after, for example, an augmentation-mastopexy operation, irradiation, or excessive scar retraction.

### 2.1.2	Shortage of Conus

As explained above, the tubular breast deformity is the most important reason for congenital double bubble deformity.

Iatrogenic reasons for a double bubble deformity can also be an excessive removal of glandular tissue after breast conservative surgery for breast cancer or over-resection of glandular tissue in breast reduction or mastopexy procedures.

### 2.1.3	Distortion by the Pectoral Muscle

A very particular but frequent cause for double bubble deformity presents itself after previous breast augmentation surgery. I any case where the origin of the pectoral muscle is cut in its lower portion, the edge of the transsected muscle shifts upward to a certain degree no matter if there was a dual-plane dissection or not. The free edge then adheres to the backside of the gland a few centimeters above the level of the inframammary crease. Depending on the degree of internal scarring, the number of fibrous ligaments between the posterior fascia of the mammary gland and the skin, the amplitude of motion of the pectoral muscle, and finally laxity of the overlying glandular tissue and skin envelope, it may be possible that a *dynamic double bubble* is formed with each contraction of the pectoral muscle. In this situation the double bubble deformity is not visible in resting position. But in some cases with more tension of the pectoral muscle on the gland the deformity may also be visible in a resting position.

2.2 Treatment

In many instances the treatment of a condition is doing exactly the opposite of what has created the deformity.

2.2.1 Adding to the Skin Envelope

When the patient is happy with the volume she has—but not with the shape of the double bubble deformity—we need to explore the possibilities to add more skin in the area between the nipple-areolar complex and the existing inframammary crease, under the condition that the inframammary crease is in the right position.

Skin envelope can be added by either stretching it through tissue expansion or adding skin by means of an autologous (free) flap. The latter is only done in cases of breast reconstruction and/or radiotherapy to the breast. Loco-regional skin flaps come in very handy here.

If there is insufficient laxity of the skin envelope and a good shape cannot be acquired by remodeling the remainder of the breast gland, one must consider introducing a breast expander in the lower quadrants. I can use a small round expander that I position very low but mostly I prefer using a croissant expander that I place pre-pectoral, just above the inframammary crease with open side cranially. This will give me a nice differentiated expansion of the lower poles only, just what I need to expand the skin. After a period of a few weeks of progressive overexpansion, I will leave the expander in place until tissue memory has disappeared. Then we will either introduce a permanent implant combined with lipofilling (technique of composite breast augmentation) or completely replace the expander by lipofilling if the remaining volume of the expander is less than 150 mL.

2.2.2 Reducing Skin Above the Double Bubble Deformity

In situations where the inframammary crease is in the right position and there is an excess of skin and gland above the double bubble deformity, it might be indicated to reduce the skin envelope just above the double bubble deformity in a vertical direction by classical mastopexy (±reduction) techniques. The advantage is that very often the scar can be limited to a vertical scar.

2.2.3　Lowering the Inframammary Crease

When the inframammary crease is too high and the distance between the nipple-areolar complex and inframammary crease is too short, expansion of this area needs to be achieved. The best surgical technique can vary a lot and can be very personal. If there is sufficient laxity of the skin envelope, lipofilling and subcisions of the area around (above and below) the inframammary crease can be effective. Repeating lipofilling and subcisions once or twice may just give you the result the patient desires. But if this area is too tight, expansion of this area both in a horizontal and vertical direction is necessary. The lower border of the capsule of the tissue expander can later serve as the new inframammary crease, if you have placed the tissue expander precisely in the right position, or it can serve as source of capsular flaps that can allow you to fix the new inframammary crease in its new position.

2.2.4　Add Volume to the Conus

When there is sufficient skin envelope available and the double bubble deformity is created by insufficient volume of the conus in the area between the nipple-areolar complex and the inframammary crease, the solution lies in adding volume in that area. This can be done by means of foreign bodies like implants or tissue expanders, or autologous tissue like lipofilling or (free) flaps. Loco-regional glandular flaps may be very convenient if sufficient breast volume is present. Lipofilling has obviously become very popular over the last few years and has taken over from moist of the other techniques but sometimes two or more sessions might be necessary to achieve the desired result.

2.3　Case Example

A 32-year-old nulliparous, healthy woman presents after having undergone 2 previous surgeries for a mild form of bilateral tubular breast and breast hypoplasia. The initial operation consisted out of a peri-areolar mastopexy combined with submuscular implants. In a second procedure an attempt was done to repair the inframammary crease and place the implant into a higher position.

After transecting the inframammary crease in the first operation (mainly on the left breast) and by continuous downward pressure on the implant by the left pectoral muscle, the implant has shifted downward below the level of the left inframammary crease. This caused significant pain complaints. The transected and shifted origin of the distal part of the pectoral muscle, stuck to the backside of the memory gland, creates the double bubble deformity that is even more accentuated with active contraction of the pectoral muscle.

Fig. 2 Oblique views of the pre-operative status of this case study

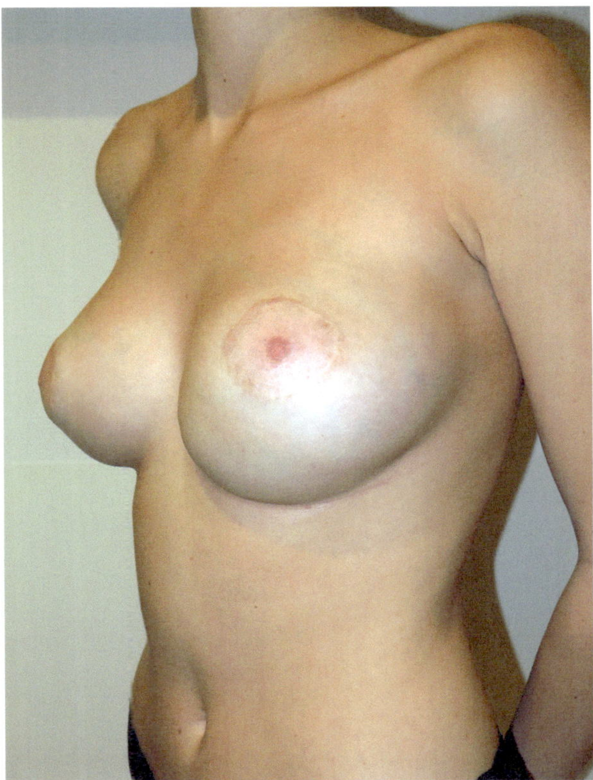

Analysis of the Problem (Figs. 1, 2, and 3):
1. Footprint: shifted downwards: Both upper mammary crease and inframammary crease are too low.
2. Conus: Total volume is correct but conus had shifted downwards.
3. Skin envelope: Expansion of the skin in the lower quadrants, caused by the implant, makes that sufficient skin is present; areola is flattened and stretched and needs correction.

Problems too correct are: (1) double bubble deformity, (2) damaged inframammary crease, (3) overextended areola, (4) unfavorable balance implant/autologous cover.

Analysis of the Surgical Approach of the Left Breast (Figs. 4, 5, and 6):
1. Footprint: The inferior border of the **footprint** of the breast was restored by direct suturing of Scarpa's fascia to the deep fascia of the intercostal muscles at the same level as the contralateral inframammary crease. The pectoral muscle was detached of the posterior fascia of the breast and repositioned into its natural position.

Fig. 3 Oblique views of the pre-operative status of this case study

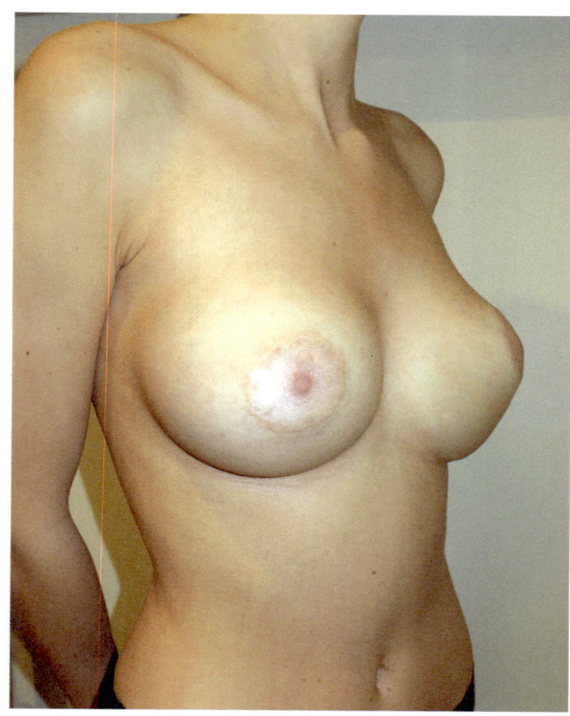

Fig. 4 Post-operative view after surgical corrections. Anterior view and oblique views

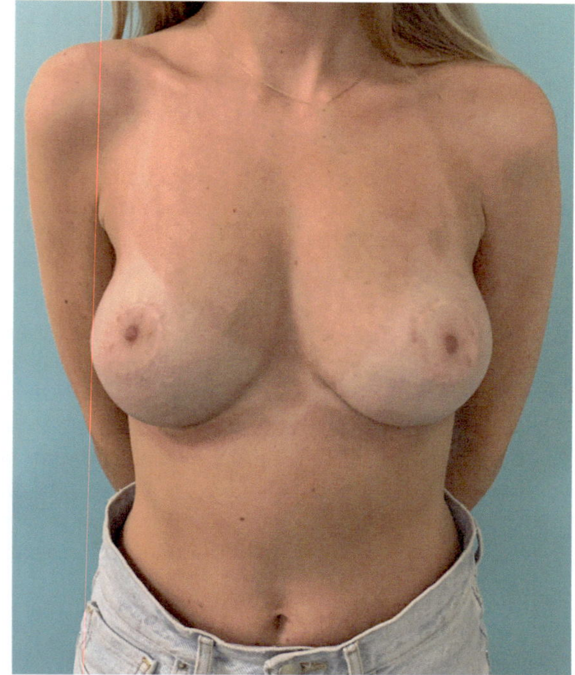

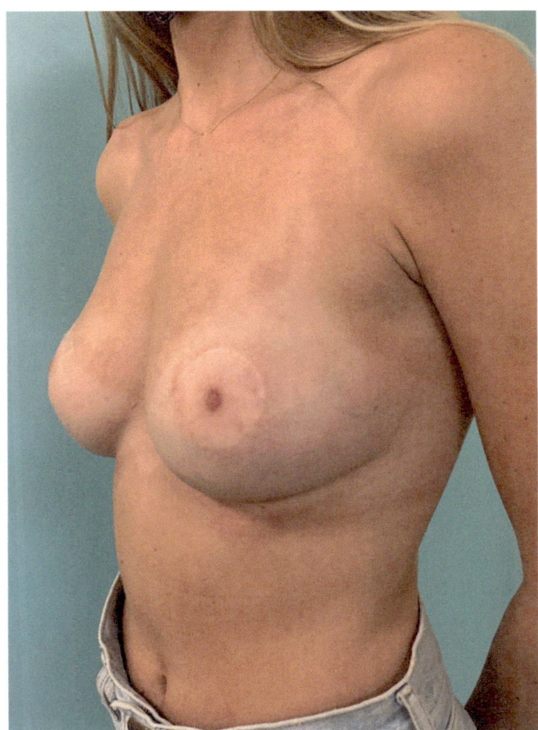

Fig. 5 Post-operative view after surgical corrections. Anterior view and oblique views

2. Conus: A new pocket was created in front of the pectoral muscle at the precise position taking into account the dimensions of the new implant (180 mL medium projection, round, nanotextured, ergonomic silicone).
3. Envelope: Thickening of the soft tissue layer by lipofilling in all 4 quadrants: reduction and subdermal reinforcement of the areola.

On the right side the existing implant was simply replaced by the same type of mammary implant as the left and lipofilling was added to the upper poles.

In a second procedure 6 months later some additional lipofilling was performed to further thicken the envelope. Final result shows a natural outcome with excellent symmetry and resolution of all pain issues.

Fig. 6 Post-operative view
after surgical corrections.
Anterior view and oblique
views

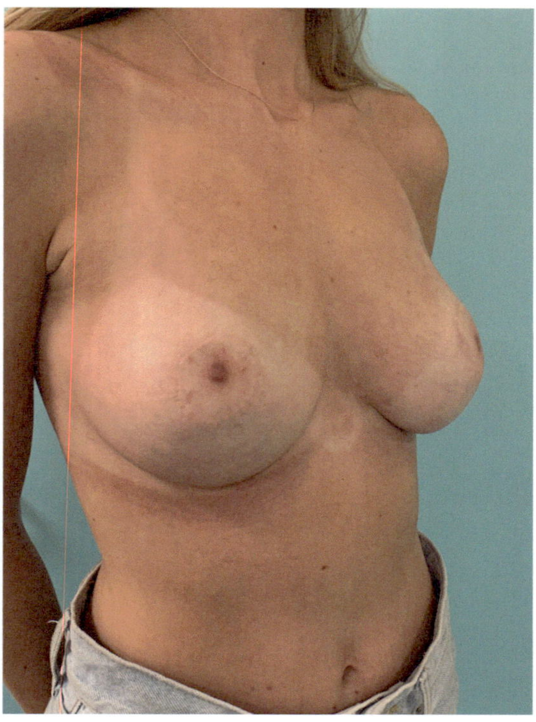

3   Wrinkling and Rippling

Wrinkling and rippling of the implant after breast augmentation is frequently observed. They are discussed together here as they often have the same etiology and they share the same therapeutical approach.

3.1   Etiology

3.1.1   Wrinkling

Wrinkling is a condition where one or more folds in the outer shell of the implant become visible or palpable through the skin. In the first phase, these sharp and pointy folds become progressively more palpable regardless of the thickness of the soft tissue envelope that covers the implant. Over time and specially when the soft tissue coverage becomes thinner, these folds even become visible.

Wrinkling of an implant starts when the inner surface of the peri-prosthetic capsule becomes smaller than the outer surface of the implant. This may happen when a surgeon introduces an implant that is too big for the pocket that has been created. Mostly however this situation is observed in cases of capsular contracture, where the cavity in which the implant resides becomes progressively smaller and where the pressure on the implant gets increasingly higher.

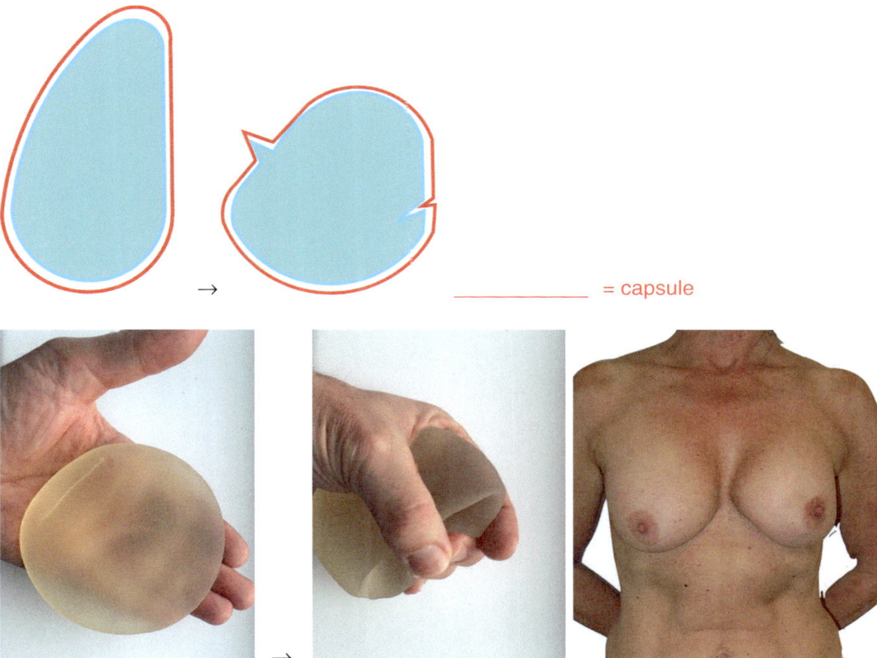

3.1.2 Rippling

Rippling is a clinical condition where a series of gentle waves are seen on the surface of the implant throughout the skin just like one would throw a stone into a pond of still water. These waves are generated by unequal forces either on the capsule or on the implant wall. In most cases actually, the implant itself is very adherent to the implant capsule and the surrounding tissues. This situation combined with a thin overlying soft tissue cover will accentuate this deformation.

Very often rippling is seen in a standing position and may disappear or shift location once the patient lays down. Because of these forces of gravity rippling is almost always seen in the upper quadrant of a breast. Rippling is also seen more frequently with water filled or under filled implants.

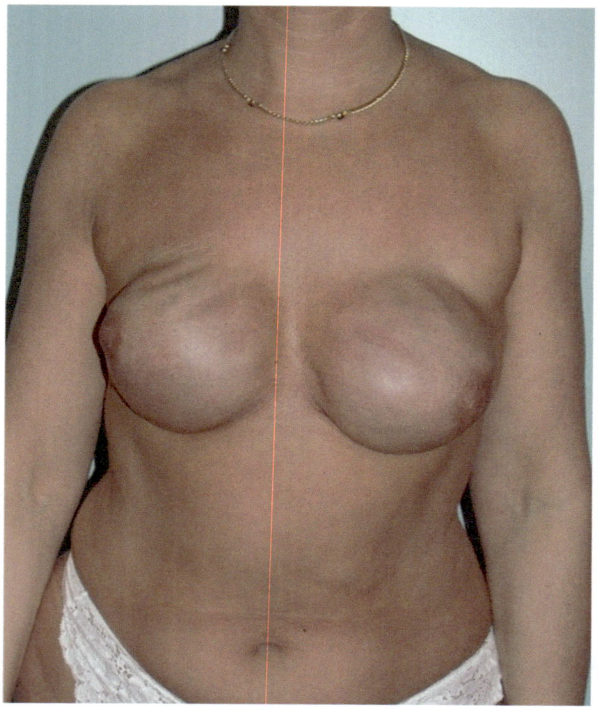

3.2 Treatment

3.2.1 Wrinkling

Theoretically, the solution of implant wrinkling lies in either making the implant cavity larger, introducing a smaller implant, or using form stable implants. If the patient insists on maintaining the same implant volume, the implant cavity can be made larger by performing capsulotomies or capsulectomies. Sometimes changing the position of the implant from a retro-pectoral to pre-pectoral position may not only allow the possibility of creating a larger implant cavity but may also offer a softer surrounding for the implants. If water filled implants were in place, one may also consider using a smaller implant eventually combined with lipofilling to compensate for the volume loss or the use of form stable implants with a more solid implant gel. Another solution may be introducing a round implant instead of an anatomical shaped implant combined with lipofilling to improve the shape of the breast (composite breast augmentation technique). If wrinkling is combined with a thin soft tissue envelope one should increase the thickness of peri-prosthetic autologous tissue layer.

There are several ways to make the soft tissue envelope that covers the implant thicker. Moving the implant to a retro-pectoral position may be helpful or the implant can be covered by an acellular dermal matrix, autologous fat or in exceptional situations by a (free) flap. Acellular dermal matrices are not only expensive, they also provide a fairly thin additional layer over the implants. They may help to reduce the occurrence of severe capsular contraction but also complications with acellular dermal matrices have been reported in variable degrees. The most common way to increase the soft tissue envelope is by the technique of lipofilling. Fat can be injected throughout all four quadrants in a subcutaneous position and can be used to modify and improve the shape of the breast.

3.2.2 Rippling

The solution to implant rippling is very similar to the solutions for implant wrinkling. If water filled implants are used, it is important to have them fully filled. Much better however is using cohesive gel implants that are form stable. Very often however these are just temporary solutions. The only solution with long-term stability is increasing the thickness of the soft tissue layer that covers the implant. Techniques on how to make the soft tissue layer thicker have been described above.

Long-term stability of a breast augmentation or a breast reconstruction with implants is directly determined by the relationship between implant size and the thickness of the soft tissue coverage. The smaller the implants and the thicker the soft tissue coverage the more long-term stability of the aesthetic result is observed. Large implants with a thin cover are prone to present with a variety of complications in the short run. Ideally a breast augmentation or a breast reconstruction is performed buy autologous tissue only.

3.3 Case Example

A 37-year-old woman presents after having undergone a breast augmentation with bilateral pre-pectoral, low viscosity gel implants 6 years earlier. She complains about asymmetry and rippling of the upper edge of her breast, mainly on the left side.

Analysis of the Problem (Figs. 7, 8, and 9):
1. Footprint: The borders of the footprint are generally in the right place: the angle between the breast and the thoracic wall is too sharp in the medial and supero-medial part of the medial edge.
2. Conus: The mammary gland can be observed as "stuck" on top of an implant that is too wide. This is responsible for a discrete double bubble deformity on both

Fig. 7 Anterior and oblique pre-operative views

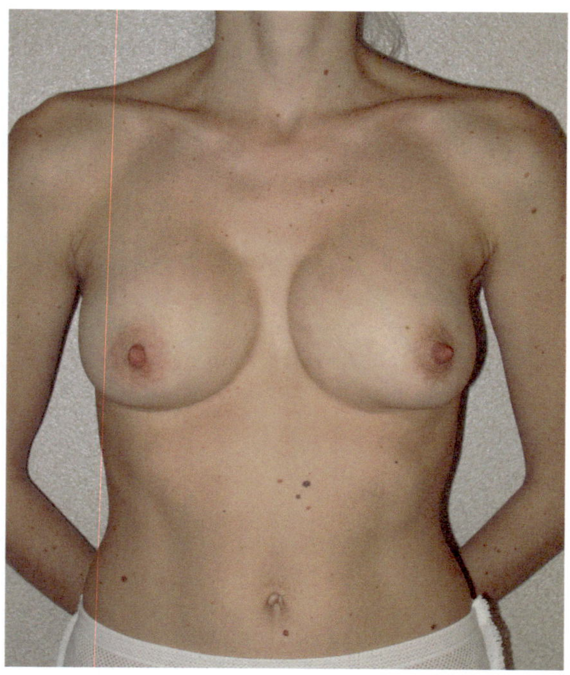

Fig. 8 Anterior and oblique pre-operative views

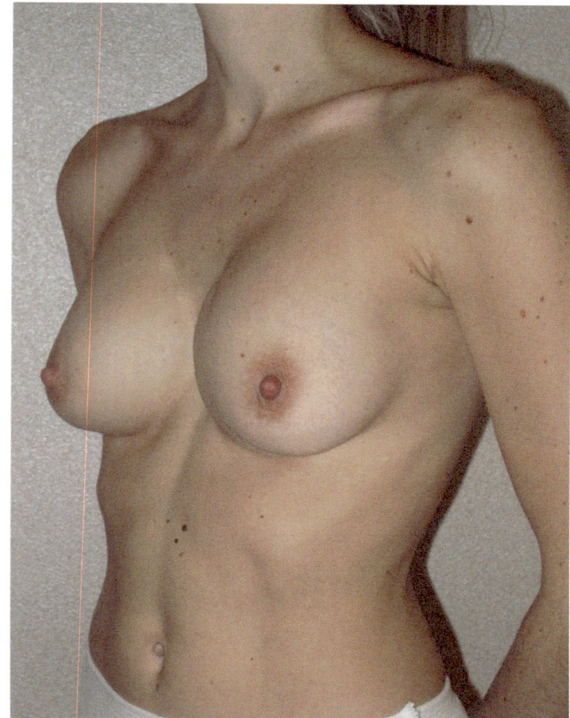

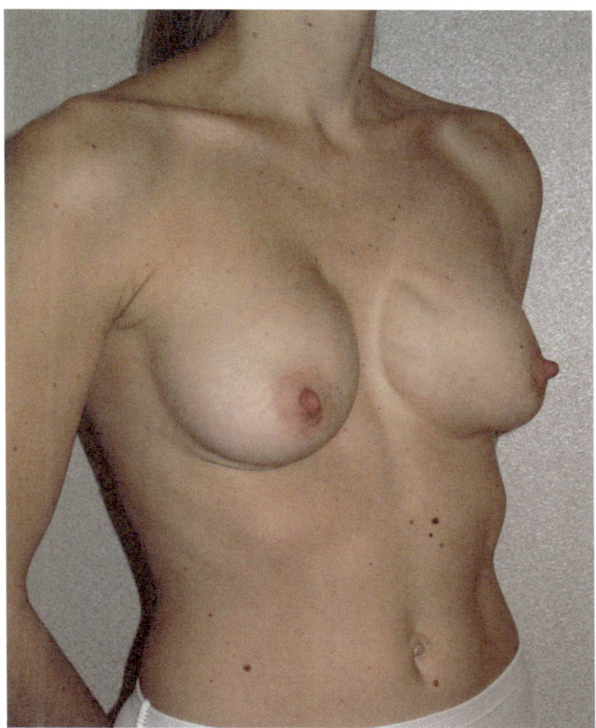

Fig. 9 Anterior and oblique pre-operative views

sides. The old inframammary crease can still be observed in the middle of this double bubble deformity.

3. Envelope: The rippling is caused by an envelope that is too thin specially over the upper poles and the low viscosity of the content of the implant. The more the implants adhere to the capsule, the more rippling will be visible.

Analysis of the Surgical Approach of the Left Breast (Figs. 10, 11, and 12):

1. Footprint: As the borders were not displaced, no corrections were necessary at this level.
2. Conus: Minimal double bubble deformities that are not caused by contraction of the origin of the pectoral muscle can easily be corrected with lipofilling. A smaller and narrower implant with an ergonomic gel was chosen to allow sufficient space for lipofilling on the edges of the footprint.
3. Envelope: The main solution of this case is thickening the soft tissue layer over the implant by lipofilling. A total of 140 ml. fat grafts was injected on each side around the existing capsule and in the subcutaneous plane.

Fig. 10 Anterior and oblique post-operative views

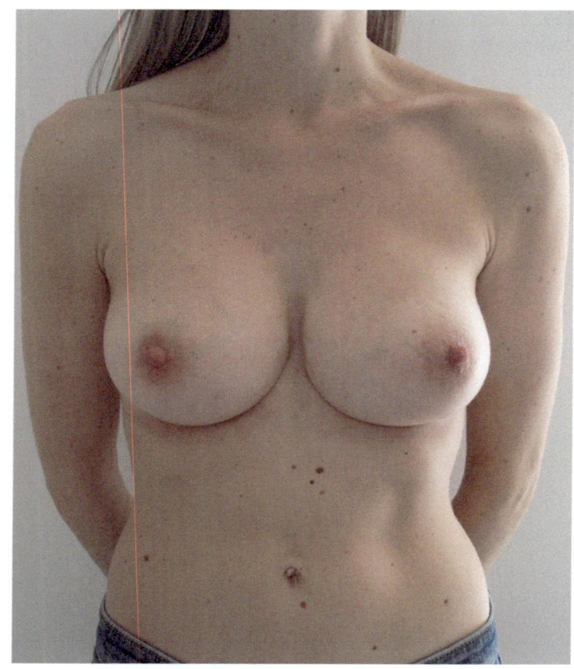

Fig. 11 Anterior and oblique post-operative views

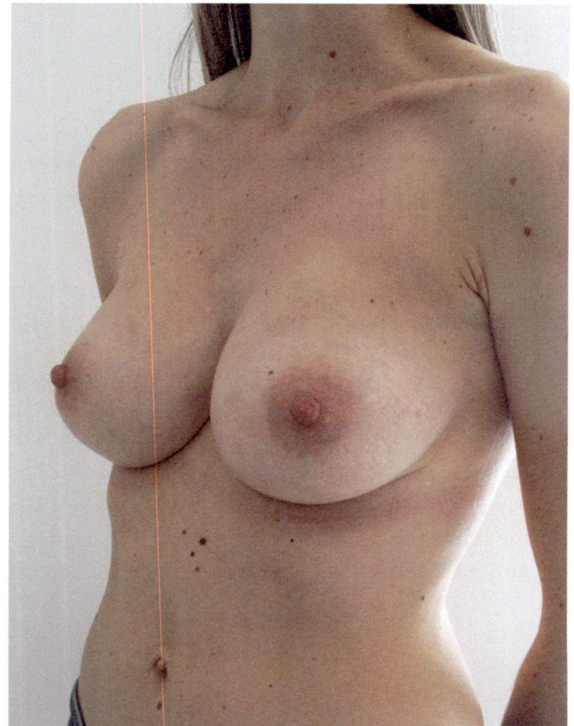

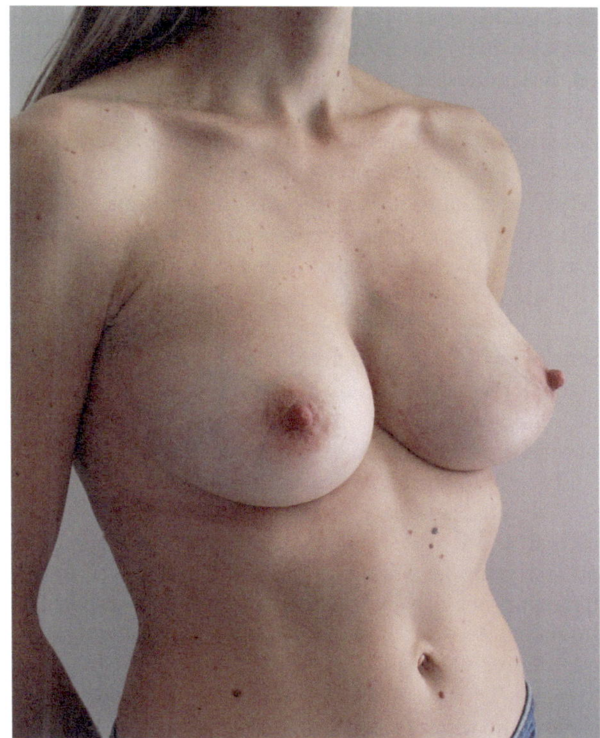

Fig. 12 Anterior and oblique post-operative views

4   Bottoming out

4.1   Etiology

Bottoming out is a clinical condition where a disproportionate large amount of mammary tissue is observed in the lower quadrants of the breast, below the nipple-areolar complex. This often leaves the upper quadrants unaesthetically flat and empty. Although bottoming out can very rarely be observed as a congenital malformation, the gross majority of patients with a bottoming out have had previous breast surgery.

There are three types of bottoming out. The first type is the one where there is an over-extension of the skin envelope, with the second one the breast conus has shifted too low over the fixed inframammary crease and in the third scenario the inframammary crease has been damaged and has descended caudally.

Type 1: footprint untouched, conus has proper shape, **skin envelope distends**

When the inframammary crease has been left untouched, bottoming out occurs because the conus has not been shaped in the right way and/or too much skin has been left in the area between nipple-areolar complex and inframammary crease. A frequent cause of bottoming out is seen after various breast reduction or augmentation-mastopexy techniques where the skin is closed with a vertical scar only. The skin and the underlying soft tissues are configured like a 3-dimensional mesh and if one only pulls in one direction, in this case tension is only been exerted in a horizontal direction, skin laxity will recur very soon after surgery as there is no tension in a vertical direction. The skin gives in, relaxes and gravity pulls the weight of the gland downward. The same will happen when an inverted-T scar is used and one does not calculate the exact amount of skin resection in the lower quadrants of the breast. After classical breast augmentation sometimes we observe excessive laxity of the skin envelope and the mammary gland causing improper descent of the implant, even when average breast implant volumes are used.

Type 2: footprint untouched, **conus too low**, skin envelope distends

Another cause of bottoming out may be the use of the wrong shape of anatomical implant with too much volume in the bottom part or just implants that are excessively large and heavy, making it impossible for the surrounding soft tissues to keep the implant in place. In autologous breast reconstruction bottoming out can be observed when the flap has not been shaped in the right way.

Type 3: **lower footprint damaged**, conus too low, skin envelope distends

The inframammary ligament is a very unique structure that consists of perpendicular and longitudinal ligaments that fix the skin to the thoracic wall at a very precise position. Mainly in the lateral part of the inframammary crease very strong ligaments anchored to the thoracic wall pass through and intermingle with Scarpa's fascia before extending into the dermal structures. The inframammary crease is also unique in a way that once these ligaments are cut, they are very hard or impossible to repair. Therefore, this structure must be respected at all times and only cut if there is really no other possibility.

Indications to undermine the inframammary crease are situations where the inframammary crease is congenitally been placed in a too high position making the distance between the nipple-areolar complex and the inframammary crease unaesthetically short. Tubular breast deformities may be a good example, but even without shape deformities, a reduced distance may be observed. Another indication to (partially) undermine the inframammary crease is the use of (very) large implants that exceed the borders of the natural footprint. As these implants are often also heavy and there is no solid structure left to go against the forces of gravity, these implants have a higher risk to shift caudally, creating a bottoming out deformity. Breast implants with a rough surface or implants that can be tagged to the chest wall may help prevent this downward shift.

4.2 Treatment

The solution lies again in doing the opposite of what has created the deformity. First of all and most important of all, if you do not need to cut the inframammary crease, don't do it.

In type 1 deformities it comes down reducing the excess of skin in between the nipple-areolar complex and the inframammary crease. When a vertical scar does not provide the desired result, a conversion to an inverted-T scar will often solve the problem. When the inverted-T scar reduction or mastopexy bottoms out, it suffices to remove more skin through the same scars. Patients that present with a congenital excessive laxity of the skin may be more difficult to correct. Either a certain amount of skin in between the nipple-areolar complex and the inframammary crease needs to be removed, adding more scars to that area, or downward pressure needs to be reduced by reducing the volume of the mammary gland or reducing the size of the implant that has been introduced. In severe cases the implant needs to be removed completely without replacement.

In type 2 deformities, one needs to deal with implant itself. Exchanging an anatomical implant to a round implant will automatically decrease the volume in the lower quadrants. If the implant is so big that it won't be held by the surrounding soft tissues, the implant volume needs to be reduced, even if the patient is not in favor. There is just no magic. There is no cure for gravity. Recurrence rate for bottoming out is very high if the same volume is used. As mentioned above, breast implants with a rough surface or implants that can be tagged to the chest wall may also help prevent downward shift.

If the inframammary crease has been damaged, as in type 3 deformities, one can consider restoring the inframammary crease by direct suturing to the chest wall, eventually assisted by the use of capsular flaps. Also the proper use of acellular dermal matrix or any other type of (non-) resorbable mesh may assist in re-creating the inframammary fold in the right position. This will often imply the positioning of smaller implants and the use of lipofilling.

It is just a general rule that better results can be achieved with smaller implant volumes. The relative loss of volume can further be compensated by the use of structural fat grafting. An additional advantage of lipofilling is the fact that it assists in improving the shape of the breast. Personally I have moved away completely from anatomically shaped implants and I only use round implants with an ergonomic silicone gel. The implant itself is just there to give me a basic volume and creates central projection. The additional lipofilling serves to improve the shape of the breast by creating fullness in the décolleté area and the upper outer quadrant. On top of that, the structural fat grafting helps me to achieve a better balance between implant volume and thickness of the soft tissue layer over the implant.

4.3　Case Example

A 41-year-old healthy patient presents after undergone multiple procedures to first augment her volume with a subpectoral breast augmentation and later to correct bilateral rippling and a waterfall deformity. In the last operation before presenting herself to me, she had undergone a vertical scar mastopexy, replacement of implants, and lipofilling of the upper pole.

Analysis of the Problem (Figs. 13, 14, and 15):

Fig. 13 Anterior and oblique pre-operative views

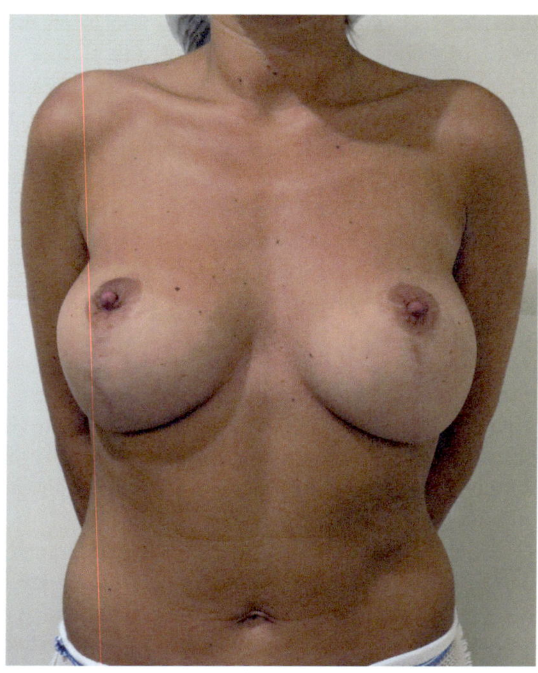

Fig. 14 Anterior and oblique pre-operative views

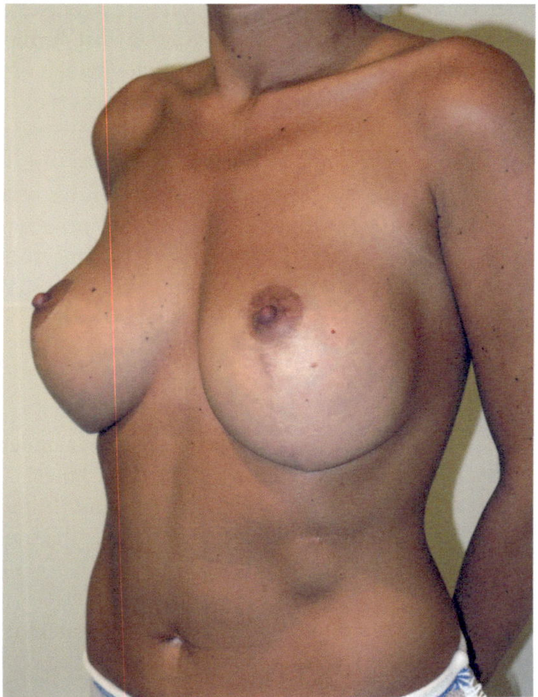

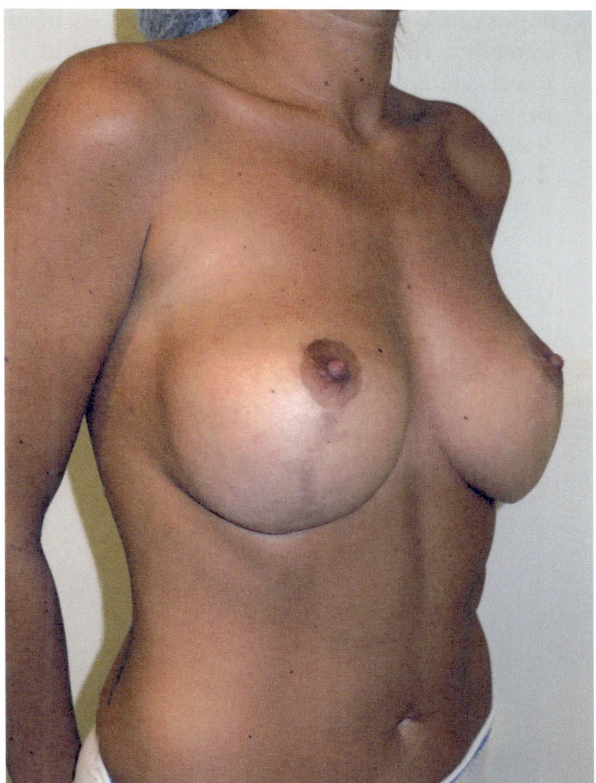

Fig. 15 Anterior and oblique pre-operative views

1. Footprint: Descent of the lower border after transection of the inframammary crease in previous procedure(s); other borders are pretty much in the right position.
2. Conus: Insufficient support of the inframammary crease (type 3 deformity) and the soft tissue envelope caused a downward shift of the conus (mainly the implant) causing bottoming out of the breast with too much volume below the equator of the breast (or the level of the nipple) and too little volume in the upper quadrants. Continuous downward pressure on the subpectoral implant by the pectoral muscle adds to the downward move.
3. Skin envelope: The reason for bottoming out was the insufficient reduction of skin and soft tissues in a vertical direction, often observed after a vertical scar mastopexy or reduction. Skin laxity was not the origin of the bottoming out in this case. An unfavorable balance between a thin soft tissue coverage and large implants deteriorates the result even more.

Analysis of the Surgical Approach of the Left Breast (Figs. 16, 17, and 18):

1. Footprint: The inferior border of the **footprint** of the breast was restored by direct suturing of Scarpa's fascia to the deep fascia of the intercostal muscles at the normal level of the inframammary crease; the origin of the pectoral muscle was resutured in its natural position. A new pocket was created in front of the pectoral muscle following the dimensions and correct position of the new mammary implants (300 mL ergonomic round, moderate projection nanotextured implants).
2. Conus: Placement of a smaller implant in the right position, supported by a solid inframammary crease and a tighter and thicker skin envelope.

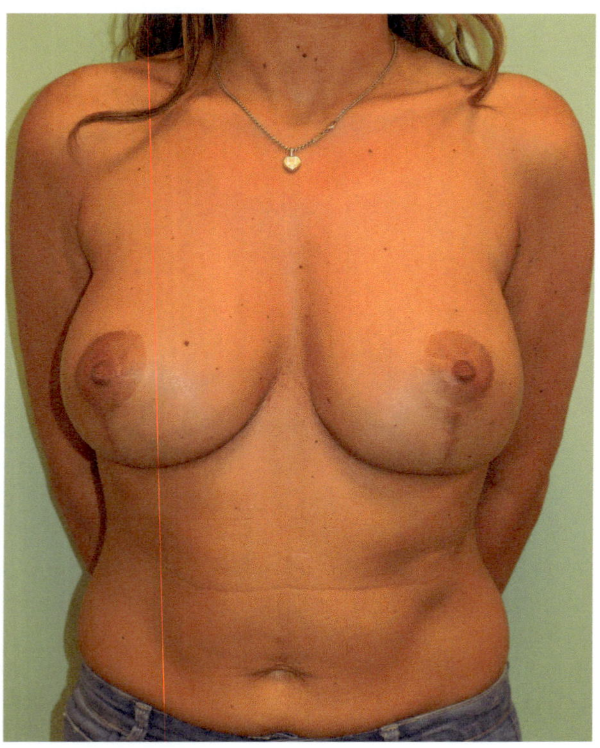

Fig. 16 Anterior and oblique post-operative views

Fig. 17 Anterior and oblique post-operative views

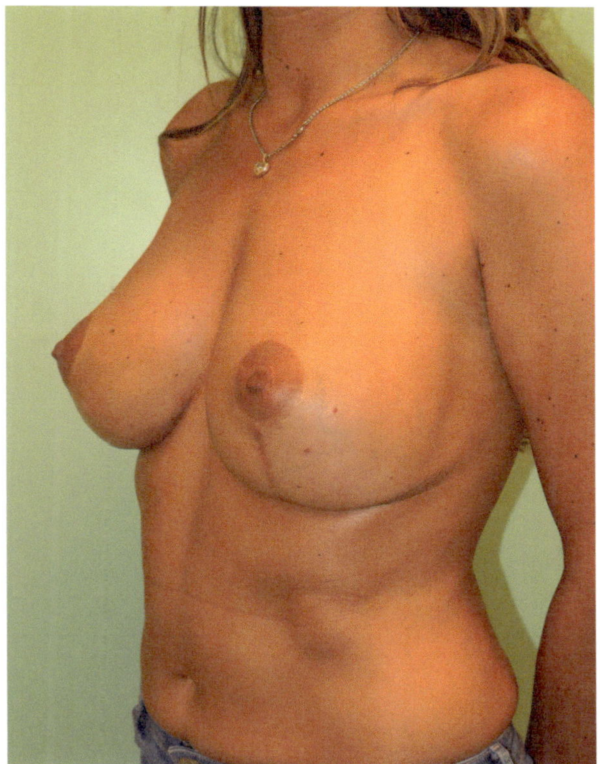

3. Envelope: Reduction of the skin excess in the lower poles by transferring the vertical scar skin resection pattern into an inverted T-scar pattern, hereby mainly reducing skin in a vertical direction; improvement of the implant/soft tissue balance by lipofilling (in total 150 mL per side) throughout the 4 quadrants of the subcutaneous layers of the breast envelope.

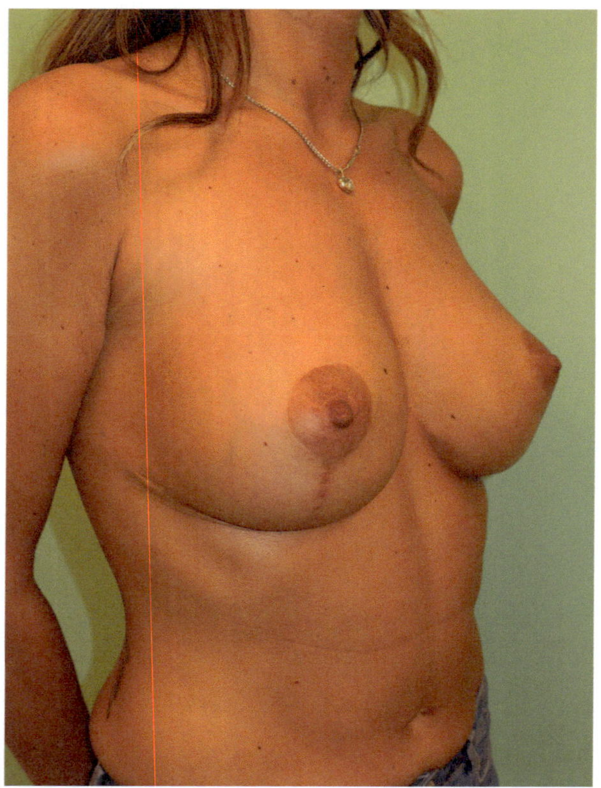

Fig. 18 Anterior and oblique post-operative views

5   Conclusion

The complications after breast augmentation discussed above are very often the result of a poor balance between the size of the implant and the soft tissue that covers the mammary prostheses. Damage to the inframammary crease is another important cause of poor results. Improving the balance between implant size and autologous tissue is an easy way to find a solution for these problems.

The three-step principle is a very easy tool in a first phase to analyze complex malformations after aesthetic and reconstructive breast surgery. In a second phase, it is an easy way to come up with a solid surgical strategy in order to correct these complications.

Disclosure I receive no financial support from any company relevant to the writing of the content of this chapter.

References

1. Blondeel PN, Hijjawi J, Depypere H, Roche N, Van Landuyt K. Shaping the breast in aesthetic and reconstructive breast surgery: an easy three-step principle. Plast Reconstr Surg. 2009;123:455–62.
2. Blondeel PN, Hijjawi J, Depypere H, Roche N, Van Landuyt K. Shaping the breast in aesthetic and reconstructive breast surgery: an easy three-step principle. Part II—breast reconstruction after total mastectomy. Plast Reconstr Surg. 2009;123:794–805.
3. Blondeel PN, Hijjawi J, Depypere H, Roche N, Van Landuyt K. Shaping the breast in aesthetic and reconstructive breast surgery: an easy three-step principle. Part III—reconstruction following breast conservative treatment. Plast Reconstr Surg. 2009;124:28–38.
4. Blondeel PN, Hijjawi J, Depypere H, Roche N, Van Landuyt K. Shaping the breast in aesthetic and reconstructive breast surgery: an easy three-step principle. Part IV—aesthetic breast surgery. Plast Reconstr Surg. 2009;124:372–82.

Implant Complications: Implant Rotation and Waterfall Deformities

Per Hedén

1   Introduction: General Reflection on Complications

Secondary breast augmentation cases are commonly more complicated than primary. These secondary procedures are frequently results of complications but can also relate to implant exchange for other reasons such as ageing of implants. In both of these circumstances, change of implant type and size is frequently considered and a similar type of surgical technique may be used if the envelope is accurately filled (see "Q2" below).

Complications after breast implant surgery can be classified in different ways:

(a) When they occur; *immediately* at the time of surgery, *early* after the first couple of days or a *late onset*.
(b) Another way of classifying complications is in relation to the *duration*, which could be *short, long-lasting or permanent*.
(c) Complications can also be *mild, moderate or severe* or
(d) Relate to *aesthetics* or *medico-functional* problems or a *mix* of these two situations.
(e) Finally it is also possible to group problems in relation why they occurred—due to *wrong implant selection*, to *faulty planning, poor surgical technique* or *wrong postoperative management.*

When it comes to aesthetic complications, these could relate to having a dissatisfied patient or a poor aesthetic result. These two situations do not always co-occur;

Supplementary Information The online version of this chapter (https://doi.org/10.1007/978-3-030-86793-5_4) contains supplementary material, which is available to authorized users.

P. Hedén (✉)
Karolinska Institute, Stockholm, Sweden
e-mail: per@drheden.com

thus a dissatisfied patient could have an objectively good aesthetic result and a patient with a poor aesthetic result could still be satisfied with the outcome. Patient dissatisfaction can usually be avoided by, bedside the use of a proper technique for selection of implant and surgery, to select the "right" patient and document (e.g. detailed phopography) the before and after situation properly. The key to success in all aesthetic treatments is to have a well-informed patient with realistic expectations. It is wise to remember that; *the reputation of plastic surgeons depends more on the patients he or she selects not to operate rather than the ones he or she actually treats.* This is especially true in the social media influence of today, where a dissatisfied patient can destroy much more of a physicians reputation that what a happy and satisfied patient builds. There are four personality types of patients that the author would recommend all physicians to be careful with when it comes to performing aesthetic treatments:

1. Patients who do not understand that exact symmetry and detailed result can not be guaranteed are more likely to be dissatisfied. All patients must understand that even if a plastic surgical procedure is millimetre exact this is not the case with the final result after healing and that the goal should instead be a great general improvement of the situation. Patients must understand that there is always a certain amount of biological variability and that this affects the healing phase and the final result.
2. Other patients to be aware of are those who do not listen and take in the information that you provide. If they have a complication such as capsular contracture, they may be very dissatisfied as they have not understood or listened to the information about the possible risk for this. If they are well aware of the fact that you have a certain risk % for a certain complication, they are more prepared to deal with this problem. It is wise to control during the consultation that the patient has understood the information provided by the surgeon by giving them some control questions.
3. Patient who describes minor defects as horrible should also be avoided. It is good to penetrate the history of how a patient is affected by an "aesthetic defect". If they spend hours in front of the mirror to look at the "defect" and avoid social encounters because of it, they may very well suffer from BDD (Body Dysmorphic Disorder). It is estimated that approximately 6% of plastic surgery patients have BDD [1]. These patients should not be operated and preferably referred to cognitive therapy instead.
4. It is also very wise to be careful with patients who are extremely disappointed and complaining about treatments done by other physicians. Even if the result after previous surgery by other physicians is objectively poor, the personality and complaints of these patients should carefully be considered when deciding to perform surgery or not. Even if you as a physician perform a good surgical secondary surgical procedure that clearly and objectively improves the situation, there is a high risk that you will be the next person on this patient's "hate list" because of the complaining personality of the patient.

If patients are selected avoiding these types of patients, the chances for a good outcome is much higher, and even if there is a complication, the chances of successful treatment of these complications are much higher. In this chapter the problems of implant rotation and waterfall deformity will be discussed.

2   Rotation of Breast Implants

Obviously, rotation of breast implants is a problem that mainly relates to anatomically shaped form stable implants (Fig. 1a–d). A low cohesive, non-form stable round implant can rotate freely without giving any deformities of the breast. A round but highly cohesive form stable implant can rotate without creating breast deformities. However, if such an implant flips upside down, the flat posterior part of the implant would create a clear deformity. This would not be the case with an implant with a much lower cohesivity.

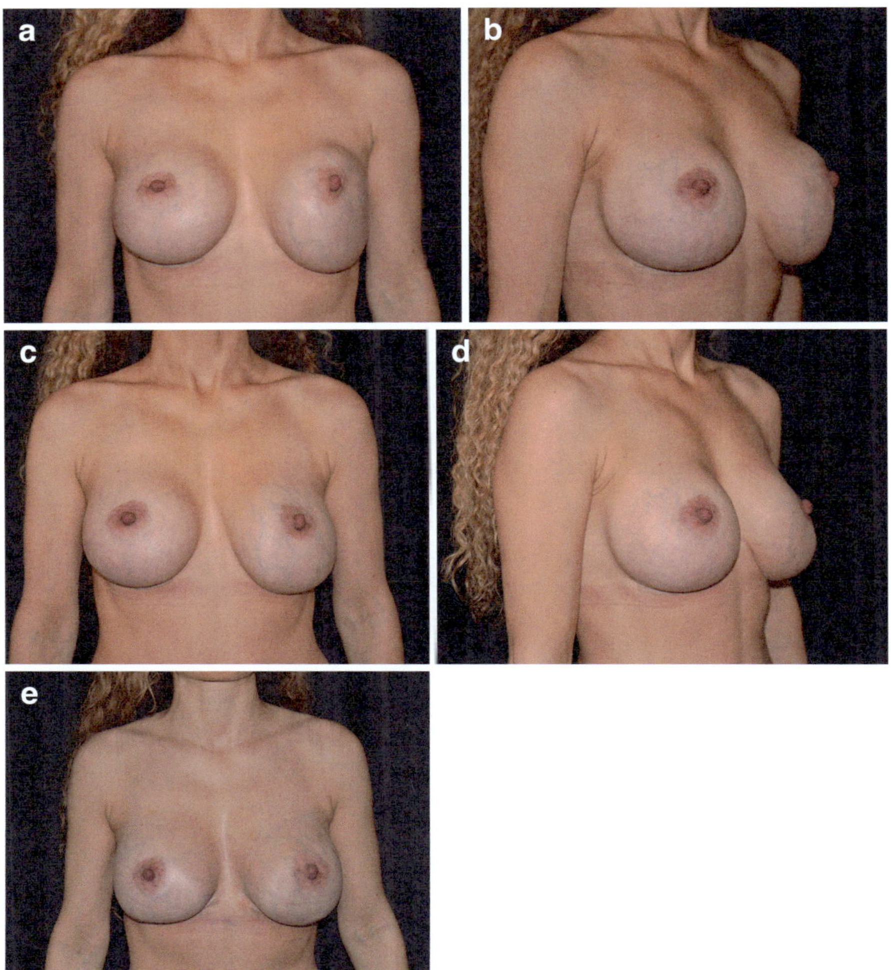

Fig. 1 (**a** and **b**) 90 degree rotation of an anatomical implant. (**c** and **d**) After manual reposition of the rotated note the implant now has an inferior malposition, this was at reoperation noted to be due to non-adhesion and double capsule formation of a macrotextured implant which makes the implants highly mobile. (**e**) After reoperation and exchange to round implants

It is also important to realise that rotation of implants is a subset of implant malposition. Thus, implant malposition could be inferior, lateral, medial, all of which creates deformities and poor outcomes after breast augmentation surgery (Fig. 2a and b). Thus, the concept of implant malposition is much larger than rotation which only is one type of implant malposition.

Implant malposition can be related to the surgical procedure, thus occurring early after surgery, but it could also occur later on when the final healing has taken place. Early implant malposition frequently depends on a poor surgical technique or preoperative planning. Thus, over-dissection of the implant pocket and poor positioning horizontally or vertically on the chest wall can produce different type of initial implant malposition including rotation. These problems can completely be avoided with a meticulous preoperative planning and surgical technique.

If implant malposition including rotation occurs late after the procedure, this frequently relates to the tissue-implant interaction. With a very thin and weak capsular formation, this do not support the breast implants and they are likely to migrate inferiorly and laterally. The risk for this problem increases with heavy implants and not using good support garments in the healing phase. Long term, the use of good support garments should also be recommended during bouncing physical activity such as jogging and trampoline jumping; otherwise the risk for implant malposition including rotation increases. The author recommended patients to wear a steady support garment day and night at least for the first three postoperative weeks and thereafter at least for 3 months when up walking, following this during physical activity with bouncing movements, e.g. running, horseback riding or jumping on a trampoline . This is especially important when using anatomical form stable implants and even more important if these are macro-textured where a strong tissue

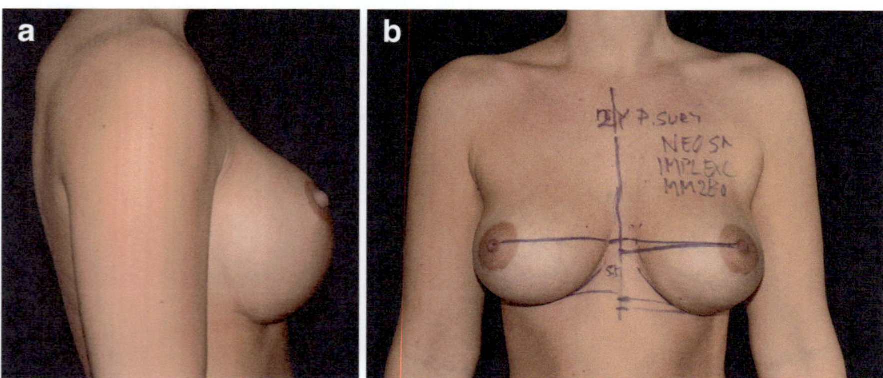

Fig. 2 (**a**) Bottom out of a smooth walled implant. No "double bubble" lower pole deformity present as the fold was poorly defined poorly defined and the glandular was minor and not dense in its nature. (**b**) Bottoming out of an anatomical implant (L side). At reoperation with a neo-submuscular pocket technique partial adhesion in the front wall of the anatomical implant prevented rotation but no adhesion/tissue ingrowth in the posterior implant surface gave the inferior malposition

ingrowth is desired. Today the Biocell® macro-textured implant is, as mentioned elsewhere, taken off the market. Many women have problems to find good support garments and recently the first underwear brands specifically developed for women with breast implants have been developed (IPOMIA.com). Seventy percent of women wear the wrong bra size according to sports biomechanist Jenny Burbage (Univ. of Portsmouth, England) and in spite of the importance of good support garments after breast augmentations most plastic surgeon have a limited knowledge about how to select the ideal bra and how this should be constructed. Many breast surgeons unfortunately also believe that all breast support garments basically are "the same", which is not true. Standard sports bras also have the wrong compression and especially anterio-posterior pressure instead of circumferential support may be wrong in these bras. Patients also usually regard medical breast support garments as ugly and when they have spent money on beautifying their breast they prefer beautiful underwear and even if the medical garment would provide the right support they commonly stop using them to early. If the importance of good support during healing and always during bouncing activities (especially true for smooth large implants) is not understood and respected, the risk for malposition including rotation of anatomical implants increases.

Plastic surgeons are in a constant battel against gravitation and tissue elasticity and besides good support garments other new technologies have been introduced to avoid implant malposition including lightweight implants (B-Lite®). The author has conducted a, not yet published, prospective study of 40 patients with lightweight implants without to date noticing any reoperations for malposition including rotations of the anatomical implants. At follow up the amplitude of implant movement during jumping up and down movement has been found to be relatively smaller when compared to traditional implants with the same volume (Fig. 3). These implants have 30% less weight in relation to their volume, which gives favourable surface area in relation to the implant weight. Data to support that this minimises malposition is still lacking but can be considered as one way of reducing risk for malposition including rotation. Other ways to minimise the risks for implant malposition is to do internal reinforcement with mesh or ADM. Synthetic absorbable meshes (e.g. TIGR® and Galaflex®) are considerably cheaper than ADM but have similar effects and are therefore favoured by many surgeons in aesthetic breast surgery (Fig. 4).

2.1   Implant Surface Technologies and Rotation

As it is likely that anatomically shaped implant would have a high degree of rotation problems if these were smooth all anatomically shaped implants have a textured surface to minimize the risk for rotational problems. A relatively new alternative to this is the use of a smooth anatomical implant with suture tabs (Truefixation®). This new concept is not yet extensively studied and no long-term data exist.

The characteristics of breast implant texturing vary greatly. The first textured implant was the polyurethane covered implant introduced in 1968 by Pangman.

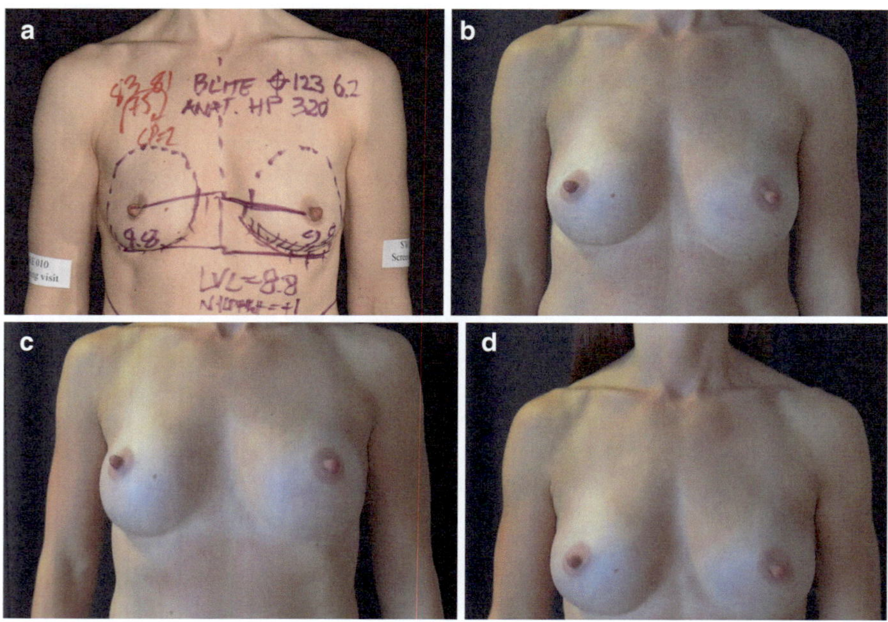

Fig. 3 (**a**) preoperative markings and planning before light weight implantation (B-lite®). (**b**) patient standing still 6 months after surgery (picture form video when patients jumps up and down). (**c**) Patient jumping up 6 months after surgery (picture form video). (**d**) Patient bouncing down 6 months after surgery (picture form video)

This resulted in a low degree of capsular contraction and therefore these implants became very popular in the 1970s. This stimulated the development of textured silicone implants. The first textured silicone implant was introduced in 1987 by McGahn (Biocell®- salt loss technology) which later on became INAMED's and it is now an ALLERGAN's implant surface technology. Due to the higher risk for BIA-ALCL (breast implant associated anaplastic large cell lymphoma) [2] this surface technology was removed from the market in July 2019. In1987, MENTOR introduced the Siltex® surface (negative PU-foam technology). A year later DOW CORNING introduced the PSI implant (laser imprint technology) which already in 1991 was taken off the market due to a high degree of seroma formation. In the twenty-first century a so-called "Nano textured" or Silksurface® (ESTABLISHMENT labs) has been introduced. This very fine texture is contrary to other textures mentioned above made on the mandrill for the implant shell which after curing is turned outside. The pore size is very small (16 µm) compared to macro-textured implants (Biocell® averaging 300 µm). This Silksurface® is classified as a smooth implant but in animal studies it has been found to behave differently as it has little macrophage infiltration which is connected to development of capsular fibrosis (Robert Langer, MIT, Boston, presented at Stockholm BTS meeting June 2018). Polyurethane covered implants have, due to low degree of malposition and capsular fibrosis, become increasingly popular in the last decade but long-term studies indicate that the

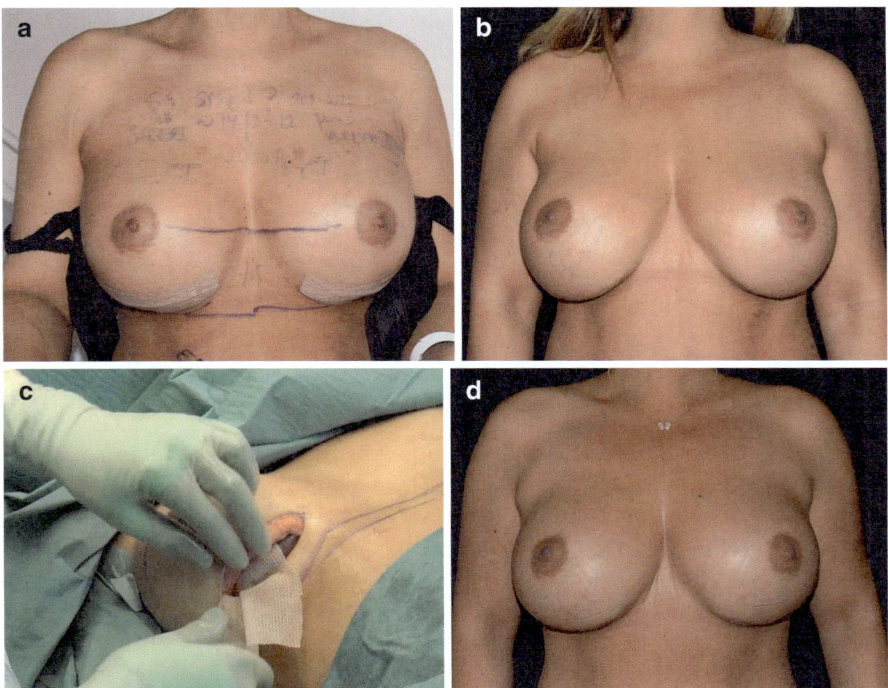

Fig. 4 (**a**) Four hour after implant exchange for a enlarged (450 cc) smooth walled implant. (**b**) Six months later with inferior malposition, very soft breasts (thin capsules). (**c**) Reoperation with mesh support (TIGR®) sutured to the border of the pectoralis muscle and swept around the lower border of the implant as an internal support. (**d**) 6 months after implantation of the mesh support

biodegradation of the polyurethane over time may reduce the long-term effects on capsular contraction [3].

With the increased focus of the aetiology of BIA-ALCL and the findings that this lymphoma "only" can occur if textured implants are used, there has been a great deal of debate on implant texturisation. Several different classification systems have been proposed [4–7]. Both the ISO 14607 system and Barr [4] classifies implant according to average surface roughness whereas Atlan [6] suggested a classification based on the surface area and Jones and Deva [5] the surface type. It has been shown that increased texturization has more bacterial contamination and that this can cause capsular fibrosis and possibly also be connected to BIA-ALCL. Considering the fact that smooth implants have more capsular contracture than smooth ones in the subglandular plane [8, 9], the issue of these problems is apparently more complex and multifactorial. Also when discussing the risk for BIA-ALCAL and smooth VS textured implants a proper risk analysis must include the mortality risk for only the surgical intervention and put this in relation to the mortality risk for having a textured implant. If smooth implants increase the risk for reoperations (e.g. because of more capsular contracture or malposition), this should be compared to the risk for mortality of ALCL. The author has, e.g. calculated that this would be equal up to 20 times higher mortality risk having a smooth implant in the subglandular plane than a textured (Siltex®) implant from the same manufacturer.

Today there is no consensus on the ideal implant surface but studies have documented that texturisation of implant surfaces reduces capsular contraction [8]. This is only documented, however, in the subglandular space where textured implants have a much lower degree of capsular contraction than smooth implants. In the submuscular space the difference in capsular contraction between smooth and textured implants is not clearly documented.

Anatomically shaped form stable implants would likely have a high degree of rotation problems if these were smooth; therefore anatomically shaped implants have a textured surface. This could be micro-textured (e.g. MENTOR CPG implants) or macro-textured (ALLERGAN Style 410 implants). There are also anatomically shaped implants with intermediate surface texturing (e.g. NAGOR and EUROSILICONE). The benefit of a macro-textured surfaces is that this can create tissue adhesion and tissue ingrowth [10]. This type of tissue adhesion is not seen with a micro-textured implant (e.g. MENTOR Siltec® surface). Thus, if an implant has very strong good tissue adhesion as would can be seen with a macro-textured implant or polyurethane surface implant, this would keep the implant in its correct non-rotated position. One could therefore assume that the risk for rotation would be lower with these types of implants than with micro-textured implants. However, this is not documented and there is really data showing that micro-textured implants rotate more than macro-textured one. Thus it appears as if the surgical technique with a snug fitting implant (*"hand in glove fit"*) pocket and a textured surface that creates friction is enough to avoid rotation of anatomically shaped micro-textured implants (e.g. MENTOR CPG implants) [9].

2.2 Anatomical Versus Round Implants

In the literature there has been a great deal of discussions related to implant surfaces and it has frequently been stated that differences in anatomically or shaped implants are minor or indistinguishable [11–13]. However, this is a great simplification as there are so many factors that influence the choice between and differences between these devices, and considering all possible pros and cons there are clear indications to use shaped implants [14]. There are basically ten different questions relating to the differences between round or anatomical implants. Publications that have stated that no difference between anatomical and round implants exists [11–13] have not considered all of the below issues:

1. *Anatomical or round shape of the implant.* It is clear that the slope of the upper pole is different between a round and an anatomical implant. This can greatly affect the appearance of the upper pole of the breast in certain situations.
2. *Implants height and width relation.* In anatomical implants the width and height ratio can be varied (full, moderate and low heights) but in round implants the

width is always equal to its height. This affects how the implant is positioned vertically in relation to the nipple areola complex (see below section on implant selection and preoperative markings) and could influence if a double bubble deformity in the lower pole is occurring or not.

3. *Implant projection* (and thus volume). The difference in the upper slope is small between a low projecting round and a low projecting anatomical implant but much larger if extra projecting implants are used. Thus, a highly projecting round implant creates a much more unnatural appearance in the upper pole than a highly projecting anatomical implant.

4. The implants position in *relation to the pectoralis muscle*. With muscle cover in the upper pole round implants are more similar to anatomical ones than if the implants are placed subglandular.

5. *Amount of glandular cover*. With thick subcutaneous tissue and glandular cover round implants are more similar to anatomical ones compared to thinner patients where the difference is much more obvious. This is especially true in more projecting implants.

6. The implants *vertical position in relation to the nipple areola complex*. If an implant is positioned high, it will give a much more unnatural pole compared to the same implant placed lower in relation to the nipple areola complex. Thus even anatomically shaped implants can create an artificial and overfilled upper pole if it is placed too high in relation to the nipple areola complex.

7. The *filling material and its cohesivity and elasticity*. Round implants with higher cohesivity and poor elasticity create more upper pole filling than implants with lower cohesivity. If the gel is very elastic (e.g. Ergonomix gel®) it will produce more lower pole volume than upper pole volume compared to high cohesive round implants with poor elasticity.

8. The *degree of implant filling*. A round overfilled, e.g. saline implant will give much more upper pole filling than a similar underfilled saline implant.

9. *Degree of capsular activity*. Capsular contraction will also contract the implant and thereby create more upper pole filling. As contracture occurs circumferentially there will also be cranial displacement of the implant and more roundness.

10. The *angle of observation*. The difference between round and anatomical implants in the anterior-posterior angle is difficult to evaluate in many situations, but if the same patient it evaluated in oblique or sideview, the difference in shape is much more obvious.

Summarising these points, the difference between round and anatomical implants cannot be too simplified as there are so many different factors influencing the final outcome of the procedure. There is without any doubt clear indication for anatomical implants and also for round implants. In modern breast implant surgery, no surgeon can use only one implant type if optimal results should be achieved. There is no doubt about the fact that there is a need for both anatomically shaped and round implants and that the selecting should be on a patient-by-patient basis based on patient preferences and the biological conditions for optimal patient satisfaction and "objective" surgical outcome.

2.3 Indications for Secondary Surgery of Rotated Implants

When does rotation of anatomical implants need secondary surgery? Obviously, the decision to correct a rotation of an anatomical implant relates to the patient's desires. Not all patients with implant rotation problems will request secondary surgery, as this may be an intermittent problem and occur very seldom. Patients may thus experience a small degree of breast deformation, which corrects itself when patients are manipulating the breast or standing in a vertical position. These patients may decide not to have secondary surgery considering the risks and drawbacks for such procedures. It is also true that rotation of an anatomical implant is much more apparent with certain shapes of implants. For instance, if a low height extra projecting implant (e.g. Allergan Style 410 LX—Low height and extra projection) rotates even a small rotation and malposition of these implants gives a very clear deformation of the breast as compared to a more round anatomical implant, especially if this is low projecting (e.g. Allergan Style 410 ML—moderate height, low projection)). Thus, some patients may have rotation without really noticing this and where there is not a clear deformation of the breast there may be no need for surgery.

2.4 Reasons and Mechanism Behind the Rotation Problem

The reasons and mechanisms behind rotation of anatomical implants is multifactorial. If an implant is correctly positioned at the time of surgery in a snug fitting implant pocket and the implants are immobilised postoperatively, the risk for rotation is minimised. However, even if these conditions are fulfilled, there is still a risk for rotation. In our own experience, using anatomical implants (Allergan Style 410) the frequency of rotational problems was minimal (0.42%) as investigated in our first series of these devices published in 2001 [15]. Over a time with increasing number of anatomical form stable implants (>40,000) with longer observation times and larger series of patients the frequency of rotational problems has increased [16]. However, these frequencies are still relatively low compared to other published frequencies [17]. It is important to understand that when a form stable anatomical implant is used, older traditional surgical techniques cannot be employed. Everything is basically different when using a form stable implant compared to the traditional techniques for implants used in the 60s, 70s and 80s. Thus, the selection process has to be differentiated, the preoperative markings are different, the surgical technique is different, and the postoperative management should be different. The fundamental importance of correct implant selection outlined below under the waterfall deformity is of great importance and the same principles when selecting implants are used when performing preoperative markings. In the surgical technique, it is recommended to be performed this through a submammary fold incision creating, in the majority of cases, a dual plane position even though subfascial and subglandular position also can be used. The pocket for a dual plane position of implant should be snug fitting and proactive haemostasis used. Thus the dissection is done with electro cautery minimising any oozing and bleeding. Leaving the loose areolar layer of tissue on the ribs and avoiding blunt dissection also minimises the risk for seroma formation and non-adhesion of an anatomical implant. One possible mechanism behind rotation is biofilm formation and the risk for this could be minimised if the recently published 14-point program is employed [18]. A strict sterile environments and surgical technique, and a meticulous pocket dissection is likely to minimize the risk for rotation of implants. Another reason for rotation of implants is formation of a so-called double capsule. The clinical appearance of this is a strongly adherent capsule on the surface of a macro-textured implant that had separated from outer layer of capsule. Thus, there are two layers of capsule, one which is adherent to the implant and another capsule attached to the gland and surrounding tissue that is separated from the double capsule. Double capsules can only occur on implants which have tissue adhesion and tissue ingrowth; thus, there has to be a pore size of the texturing >150 μm [10]. If a micro-textured implant is used, there is no tissue ingrowth into the surface of the implant and thus double capsule formation is unlikely if even possible. The mechanism behind double capsule formation is not clear but in the experience of the author it is common to see partial double capsule of the posterior side of macro-textured implant close to the smooth patch of the implant. The ventral side of a macro-textured implant is usually adherent and attached to the gland but if this ruptures the implant can start to rotate. If a true double capsular formation is created circumferentially around an implant, this creates a very smooth surface which facilitates rotation and is usually a situation which needs secondary correction.

2.5 Surgical Correction of Rotation

There are multiple different options to treat implant rotation where one straightforward and simple alternative could be to change implants to low cohesive round devices, which cannot create the typical rotated deformity of the breast. However, rotation is frequently unilateral, and many patients are happy with the contralateral breast. To only exchange one implant to a non-form stable round device can create asymmetry and is not advised in the majority of cases. Most patients would need bilateral implant exchange in these situations, and if patients are happy with the breast that does not rotate, it is usually better to address the rotated side with the same type of implant that the patient has on the non-rotated side. Since July 2019 Style 410 implants with Biocell® surface technology is no longer on the market and a decision has to be made of having different implants on each side or changing both implants even if the patient is happy with one side. One solution could be to find an implant that has similar dimensions as the no longer available Style 410 implant. Example of this is the Style 410 MM280 model which has very similar dimensions as the CPG 321280 implant. When treating a rotated implant unilaterally it is strongly advised to change the implant, as biofilm formation [5] may be one of the causes for rotation. This cannot be washed away from the implant surface and thus the implant has to be changed. To insert a new implant in the same pocket is neither advised as this increases the risk for rotation even if a capsulorrhaphy is used to minimise the size of the pocket. In these cases, it is instead recommended to create a new pocket. If implants are subglandular, a capsulectomy and capsulorrhaphy can be performed but more commonly a site change to a submuscular position is recommended. This can easily be performed but by standard dual plane elevation of the pectoralis muscle. Usually only a capsulectomy of lower pole of the subglandular pocket is needed in these cases. Note that the elevated pectoralis muscle should be attached to the overlying gland to minimize the risk for luxation of the implant into its original subglandular position.

If the rotated implant is in the submuscular position, site change to a new subglandular-fascial pocket could be considered. However, many of these patients have muscle cover for a reason (e.g. they have thin coverage and risks for rippling and implant visibility) and the neo-submuscular pocket technique is the recommended method instead.

The author developed the neo-submuscular pocket technique in the 1990s, and presented for the first in 1998 (*"Secondary new submuscular technique* "Stanford Hospital Breast meeting, London) and later on in several international meetings. The technique was never published by the author but later described by Maxwell and Gabriel [19]. The surgical techniques involve dissection via the previous, usually sub-mammary fold scar, to the thoracic fascia following this in a proximal direction until the capsule is exposed. The capsule is then followed with the implant in place to create a supracapsular plane of dissection. This dissection is carried on as far as possible but when the vertex of the implant is reached the dissection becomes increasingly difficult. At this stage, the capsule is opened, and the implant is removed which deflates the implant capsule and makes dissection much more difficult if the capsule is not stretched. To facilitate this dissection two vascular clamps are attached to the capsule and the capsule is stretched. This makes the dissection much easier and the dissection is carried on in a cranial direction, in the direction of the sternal notch. Depending on which type of muscle division that has been done in the previous procedure the height of the muscle border can be at different levels. When the muscle border is approached, dissecting with an electro cautery on top of the capsule, it is easily diagnosed by the twitching of the muscle. The muscle border is elevated, and a plane is created deep to the muscle on top of the capsule. If the capsule is thin, this dissection is somewhat more difficult but in the majority of cases it is an easy and bloodless field to dissect in. After having dissected underneath, the border of the pectoralis muscle for a couple of centimetres the dissection is usually very easy to carry on with either an electro cautery or a pair of scissors. The height of the pocket is carefully measured during the dissection to avoid over-dissection. The width of the pocket is thereafter carefully expanded so the pocket is not over-dissected. Remember that the underlying capsule will be kept in place and the ventral leaf of the capsule will further increase the size of the new pocket created on top of the capsule. Therefore, check the width very carefully and this could be one indication to use a sizer, possibly even using the old implant as a sizer in this new pocket to see that it is not over-dissected. The final part of the dissection, which is most difficult, is the medial dissection along the sternal boarder and the inferior medial origin which should not be dehisced from the sternum.

Usually the neo-submuscular plane of dissection is bloodless and easily performed. When the pocket has been created it is advised to place a drain in both the posterior capsule and the neo-submuscular plane. Thus, the drain goes through the two pockets. The capsule is then left behind as the posterior wall of the new pocket and the incision in the capsule is closed. The author favours use of a running barbed Monoderm 2/0 suture, which can also be used to anchor the two leaves of (the anterior and posterior) capsule to each other. In a situation where the neo-submuscular pocket technique is used to correct a too high positioned implant (as exemplified below in water fall deformity) the posterior and ventral leaf of the old capsule pocket can be left without suturing them together which facilitates movement of the implants in their new neo-submuscular pocket position. This will then act as a gliding surface against the rib cage and let the breast implant settle in a more natural way in spite of the fact that it has a snug fitting implant pocket on top of the old pocket. After recreating the submammary fold, suturing the Scarpa's fascia to the thoracic fascia using a running number 0 Quill suture, the superficial layers are closed with deep dermal relaxing ridging sutures and a running subcuticular intradermal stitch. Usually two layers of Monoderm 2/0 is favoured in this layer (Fig. 5 and included Video 1 demonstration of the neo-submuscular technique).

The *neo-submuscular pocket* technique is useful in a multitude of secondary procedures such as

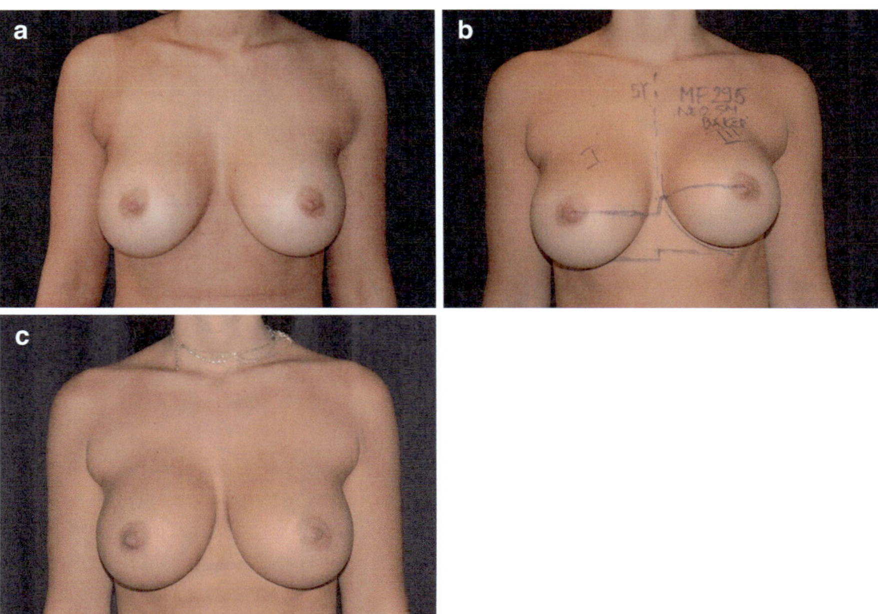

Fig. 5 (**a**) One years after insertion of anatomical implants. (**b**) Four years later with capsular contracture. (**c**) One year after reoperation with L sided neo-submuscular pocket technique and implant exchange (see Video 1)

1. Implant mal position (descent, double bubble, waterfall deformity, rotation, etc.).
2. Capsular contractions.
3. Poor muscle animation.
4. Implant visibility.
5. Implant rippling and palpability.
6. Synmastia.

When rotational problems are corrected with a neo-submuscular pocket technique, placing a new implant of the same dimensions and shape as previously used, this is successful in the majority of cases. It is however advisable that the patient is very careful with displacement during physical activity and a steady support bra is of great importance in the first couple of months after the procedure.

In *re-rotation cases* it may be wiser to change implants to round devices with lower cohesivity on both sides. When selecting implants in this situation a similar base width and volume as the anatomical device can be selected but this may increase the risk that the round implant, even if this is low cohesive, will be slightly too high positioned with to round upper pole compared to the appearance of the anatomical implant. If instead a slightly narrower implant base width is selected, a good correction can usually easily be achieved with the exchange of both implants positioned in the same pockets (Fig. 1e).

3 The Waterfall Deformity

There has been some confusion in the nomenclature of what the "Waterfall deformity" constitutes. Some physicians refer to waterfall deformity as an implant, which is too low positioned in relation to the nipple areola complex. This is according to the author not a correct definition, as this should rather be regarded as bottoming out of implant, possibly with a contour irregularity ("double-bubble") deformity. The waterfall deformity is rather an implant too high positioned in relation to the nipple areola complex, where lax breast tissue hangs like a waterfall on top of the implant.

3.1 Mechanisms and Reasons for Development of the Waterfall Deformity

If an implant is placed too high in relation to the nipple areola complex, there will be too much fullness in the upper pole of the breast and too little lower pole fullness. The aesthetic ideal of a breast is to have more volume in the lower pole compared to the upper pole [20]. If the breast tissue with its envelope is tight, there will be no Waterfall deformity, but if the breast tissue is lax and the envelope is slightly excessive, it will hang distal to the implant creating the typical Waterfall deformity. This deformity can also be caused by capsular contraction where there is a cranial displacement of the implant, especially if this is smooth where the pocket initially is relatively large. With a circumferential constriction the implant hanging in the lower

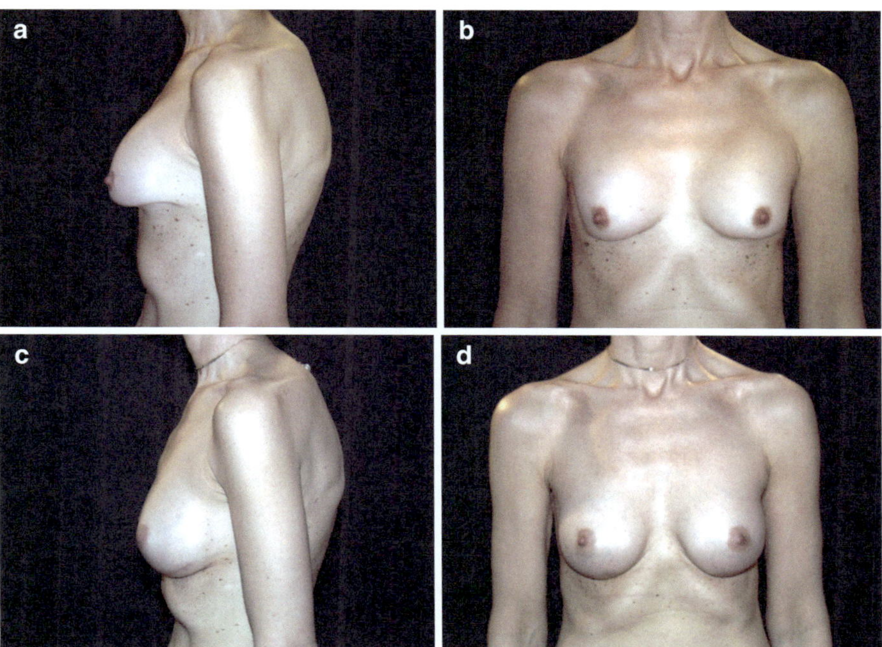

Fig. 6 (**a** and **b**) Several years after insertion of smooth walled implants (unknown surgeon)—
moderate capsular contracture. Moderate waterfall appearance due to too high positioned implants
but only moderate and tissue excess in lower pole. (**c** and **d**) After neo-submuscular pocket and
implantation of anatomical implants in a lower position. Similar degree of capsular contracture but
implants in correct position in relation to the NAC. Note that the old IMF scar has become more
visible as the nipple to scar distance was planned too short in the initial operation. If a too short
N-NIMF distance is used and attempt to suture this down to the thoracis wall is will displace the
implant in a cranial direction (see text on: Q2)

part of the pocket is cranially displaced. With well-integrated macro-textured
implants much less of this type of cranial displacement is usually occurring during
capsular contracture (Fig. 6). If no capsular contraction is present, the Waterfall
deformity can basically be completely avoided by a correct implant selection and
planning (Figs. 7, 8 and 9).

3.2 Preoperative Implant Selection and Planning to Avoid Postoperative Problems Such as the Waterfall Deformity

In the past implants were usually selected relatively arbitrary based on surgeons
experience, but in the first half of the 1990s with the introduction of anatomical
form stable devices that couldn't be squeezed into the wrong fitting implant pocket
it became necessary to plan and select an appropriate implant dimension in relation
to the biological conditions. This is now also the standard of care even if round low

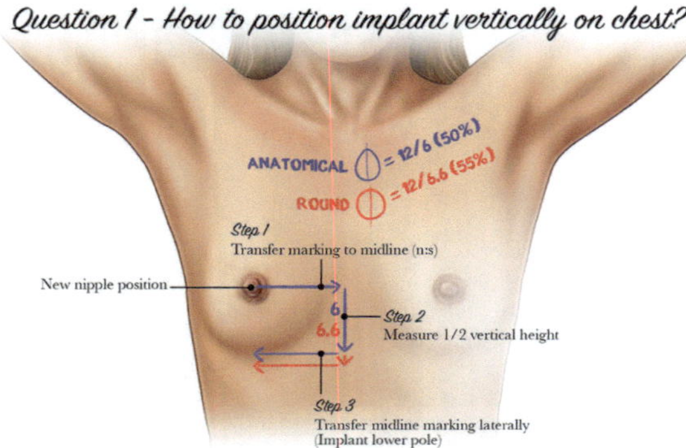

Fig. 7 Illustration to how to plan the position the implant vertically on the chest wall in relation to the NAC = Q1 in the "Q2 method". Illustration taken from the videos series *"Safe and predictable breast augmentation"* by Per Hedén—Published with permission from QMP videos (https://www. qmp.com/product/safe-and-predictable-breast-augmentation/151)

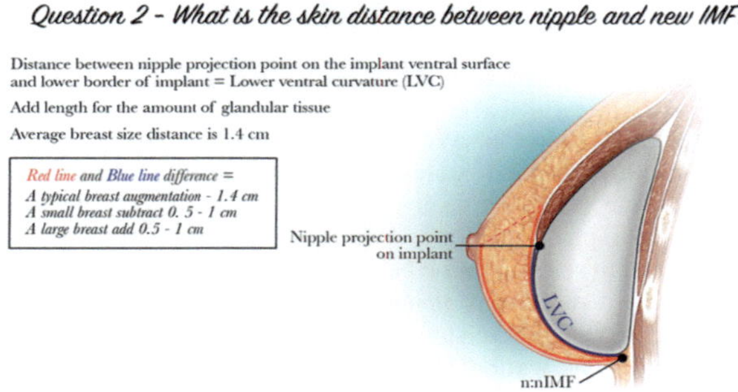

Fig. 8 Calculation of how long the distance of skin need to be in the lower pole after a breast augmentation and how this related to the LVC value and the amount of gland covering the implant in the lower pole = Q2 in the "Q2 method". Illustration taken from the videos series *"Safe and predictable breast augmentation"* by Per Hedén—Published with permission from QMP videos. (www.qmp.com)

cohesive implants are used and measurements should always be done when selecting appropriate implants. Having defined patient desires and examined the breast envelope, gland, symmetries, etc. the implant dimensions are selected. This includes selecting the right width and height of the implant and also the correct projection and shape. In the selection process the same principles as in preoperative markings should be used and *there are two fundamental questions that always should be kept in mind when selecting implants and doing preoperative markings*. The author begun to develop these principles in the second half of the 1990s and with the gradual small alterations this development can be followed in a series of book-chapters

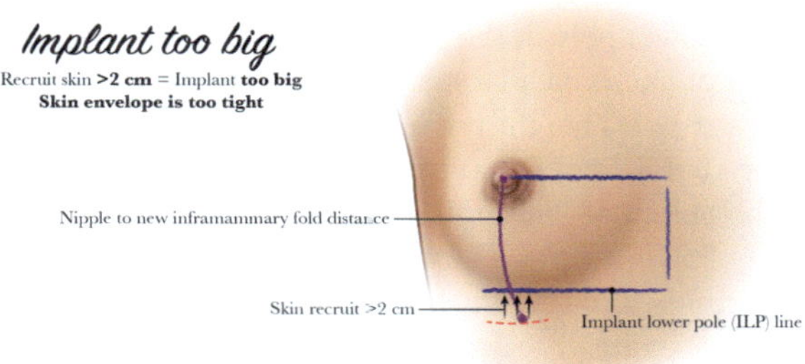

Fig. 9 If the implant is large (long LVC value) in relation to the to a tight envelope then N-NIMF distance will be distal to the ideal position of the lower pole of the implant. Illustration taken from the videos series *"Safe and predictable breast augmentation"* by Per Hedén—Published with permission from QMP videos. (www.qmp.com)

and publications [21–25]. The method has been called the Q2 method, the AK or Akademikliniken method.

Q1 The first one of these questions is: *How should the implant ideally be positioned vertically on the chest wall in relation to the nipple areola* complex? (Fig. 7).

Q2 The second important question is: *How long distance of skin will be needed between the nipple areola complex and the submammary fold?* (Fig. 8).

To answer **Q1** the author did some fundamental and important observations to answer in the late second half of the 1990s.

(a) The first observation was that *a correctly performed breast augmentation truly elevates the nipple areola complex*. This is related to volume increase in the lower part of the breast acting as a pendulum rotating the NAC outward and up. Thus the distance between the sternal notch and the nipple does not change but in relation to the fixed tissues of the midline there is a true elevation. If the breast implant is placed to high on the chest well with more filling in the upper pole the nipple elevation is counteracted.

(b) The second observation was that planning and measurements on the breast tissue was difficult as this is greatly variable when it comes to amount of gland, envelope, laxity, etc. and therefore transposing the nipple position to the midline and doing the markings and planning along the sternal midline where tissue is much more rigid is a good way of performing implant selection and preoperative marking. Thus a *nipple sternum marking is an important tool in the implant selection and preoperative planning*.

(c) The third, very important observation was that the *postoperative nipple position could be estimated with arm elevation*. Evaluating several hundred breast augmentations the author found that the correct way of predicting nipple position postoperatively was obtained by asking the patient to clasp her hands on top of the head, thus elevating the arms 45° above the horizontal plane.

Considering the aesthetic ideals of the breast [20] the goal is to have more of the implant volume in the lower pole of the breast, approximately 55%. For this the goal is to have half (50%) of anatomically shaped implants (as these have more volume distributed in the lower pole) height positioned distal to the nipple areola complex postoperatively. For round implants, especially if these are of higher cohesivity, more than half of the height of the implant should be distal to the nipple projection point (approximately 55%).

Using these principles, the first question (**Q1**) on how to position the implant vertically on the chest wall can be answered. If, for example, an anatomical implant with a height of 12 cm is to be used, 6 cm (50%) of the height should be placed distal to the nipple areola complex. The patient is asked to place her hands on top of her head, predicting the new nipple position. With this hand position the nipple position is horizontally transferred to the midline (*NS line = Nipple sternum line*) and, after lowering the hands, as much implant height desired to be distal to the NAC postoperatively is measured and marked, in this case 6 cm. The patient is then asked to elevate her hands on top of her head again and at the distal end of this midline measurement a horizontal marking is done parallel to the nipple sternum line transferring the midline marking laterally and thereby answering where the lower boarder of the implant should be placed (this is called the *ILP- line = Implants lower pole*). If a 12 cm round implant instead was used, 55% of the baseplate height should be measured distally in the midline, thus 6.6 cm (Fig. 7).

To avoid complications such as a waterfall deformity, it is also necessary to check that the amount of skin between the nipple and the implants lower pole position is filled adequately by the implant. This is the second important question to answer in any breast augmentation (**Q2**). The filling of the envelope depends on the implant dimensions and the amount of gland. The length of the implants lower ventral curvature is of great importance for this calculation. This equals the distance from the horizontal nipple projection point on the implants ventral surface down to the lower border of the implant (the so called LVC value). Obviously more projecting implant and higher base plate must have a longer distance between the nipple and the new inframammary fold; thus more skin is needed. The LVC value can be calculated for any implant and this has been performed by the author for most implant on the. The horizontal nipple projection point on the implants ventral surface varies if the implant is planned to be 50 or 55% distal to the nipple after the augmentation and thus the LVC value varies in relation to this. In addition to the LVC length of the implant the distance of skin needed between the nipple and the inframammary fold depends on the amount of covering gland. This can be adequately calculated by measuring the convexity of the breast (with hands on top of the head to simulate the nipple elevation) and then subtracting the "inside" distance between nipple projection point to the ILP line, which is equal to the half the height of the implant (if anatomical). This way of calculating how much distance that has to be added to the LVC value in relation to the amount of covering gland, however, has by many physicians been regarded as a difficult process. Because of this author introduced a simplification after evaluating several hundred augmentation patients. It could be concluded that the average length of skin that had to be added to the LVC value of the implant was 1.4 cm. Thus, new charts for different implants with the nipple to new IMF distance (*N-NIMF*) have been developed. These charts provide the N-NIMF distance for any type of implant and this distance is equal to the LVC value + 1.4 cm. Thus physicians do not have to calculate, they just look into the charts to define which distance of skin that will be needed in relation to the selected implant. To get an even more accurate distance 0.5–1 cm could be subtracted from this N-NIMF chart if the patient has a small or very small breast and alternatively in a large or very large breast 0.5–1 cm could be added.

Recently to simplify these principles even more a breast implant planner APP (available in 2021 on APPstore or Android) has been developed. This will contain a simplified description of the above principles, dimensions of all implants in the market, the calculated vertical implant position (50or 55% of height) **Q1,** and the distance of skin needed between the nipple and the postoperative IMF (nipple to new inframammary fold N-NIMF) **Q2.**

So why is it important to answer both the question on how the implants should be placed vertical on the chest wall and how long distance of skin that is needed in the lower pole of the breast? If there is a perfect match between the implant and the breast tissue including the envelope, the lower pole of the implant will be positioned exactly at the existing inframammary fold. When the skin then is fully stretched, the amount of skin in the lower pole between the nipple and the inframammary fold is equal to the nipple to new IMF distance (N-NIMF) according to the chart for the implant that has been selected. This is in the ideal world but in many situations, this is not the case. If the implants vertical position is above the amount of skin needed in the lower pole of the breast which could be the situation in a very tight envelope and a patient desires a large implant, 1–2 cm of skin could be recruited to the lower pole by making the incision distal to the implants lower border (the ILP line) (Fig. 9). This is done by suturing the Scarpa's fascia (or supra Scarpa's tissue in patients with more subcutaneous tissue) down the thoracic fascia along the ILP line. If the distance between the implants lower pole line and the amount of skin needed is more than 2 cm, the implant is too big for the envelope and a smaller implant should be recommended to the patient. In the reverse situation (usually in pseudo-ptotic breast or patient with lax tissue) the implants lower pole (**Q1**) is distal to the amount of stretched skin needed in the lower pole according to the charts as described above. The incision can then be made above the implants lower pole and dissection is carried on distally to the implant lower pole position (ILP line). The incision is then sutured down to the implant lower pole line. However, if the discrepancy between the amount of skin and the implants vertical position is more than 2 cm, there is too much laxity of the breast and more projecting implants or different shapes and sizes of implants should be considered. If not analysed and too much in the lower pole is present and not respected, this predisposes for a postoperative *Waterfall deformity*.

Alternatively to stretching the skin distally or using alternative implant dimensions and sizes is to reposition the NAC. If a mastopexy is needed and the same principles for planning is used but in a reversed fasion. Thus the IMF is used for implant lower pole position and the IMF/ILP markings are transferred to the midline and measurements are done in a proximal direction instead. Elevating the hands on top of the head the midline markings are transferred laterally to mark the new nipple position (sternum to new nipple position line S-NN). These principles where published by the author already in 2009 [26].

By analysing these two questions; **Q1** The implants vertical position on the chest wall in relation to the nipple areola complex, and **Q2** The amount of skin needed in the lower pole of the breast, most problems such as Waterfall deformity but also many other problems and complications in breast augmentation surgery can be avoided. These measurements can also be used to analyse if a mastopexy augmentation is needed or not.

3.3   Correction of Waterfall Deformities

In most situations where there is a Waterfall deformity there is too much laxity in the envelope in relation to the implant and the easiest way of correcting this is to reduce this excessive envelope and reposition the nipple areola complex (Fig. 10). If the Waterfall deformity is small, a peri-areolar procedure may be sufficient to correct it, but based on the analysis as described above a vertical or inverted T procedure may be needed.

In some situations Waterfall deformities could be corrected by placing the implant more distally doing a capsulotomy in the lower pole of the breast, but when performing these types of procedures remember that if an anatomical device has been used there is a risk for rotation; thus a neo-submuscular pocket may instead be needed. When repositioning the implant more distally it is important to analyse that the amount of skin needed in the lower pole of the breast will be accurately filled. Remember also that when placing implants well distal to an existing submammary fold there is a risk for a double bubble deformity in the lower pole of the breast. This risk increases greatly if the gland is dense and well defined. This may need fat grafting, scoring of the gland, Puckett procedures etc.

4   Conclusions

Breast implant rotations and Waterfall deformities are conditions that in the majority of cases can be avoided by meticulous implant selection, preoperative marking, correct surgical technique and good support garment postoperatively. Careful analysis of the breast including the important questions on (**Q1**) how to position the implant vertically on the chest wall and (**Q2**) amount of skin needed in the lower pole of the breast are fundamental principles that should be used in every breast augmentation patient to avoid and treat these type of problems.

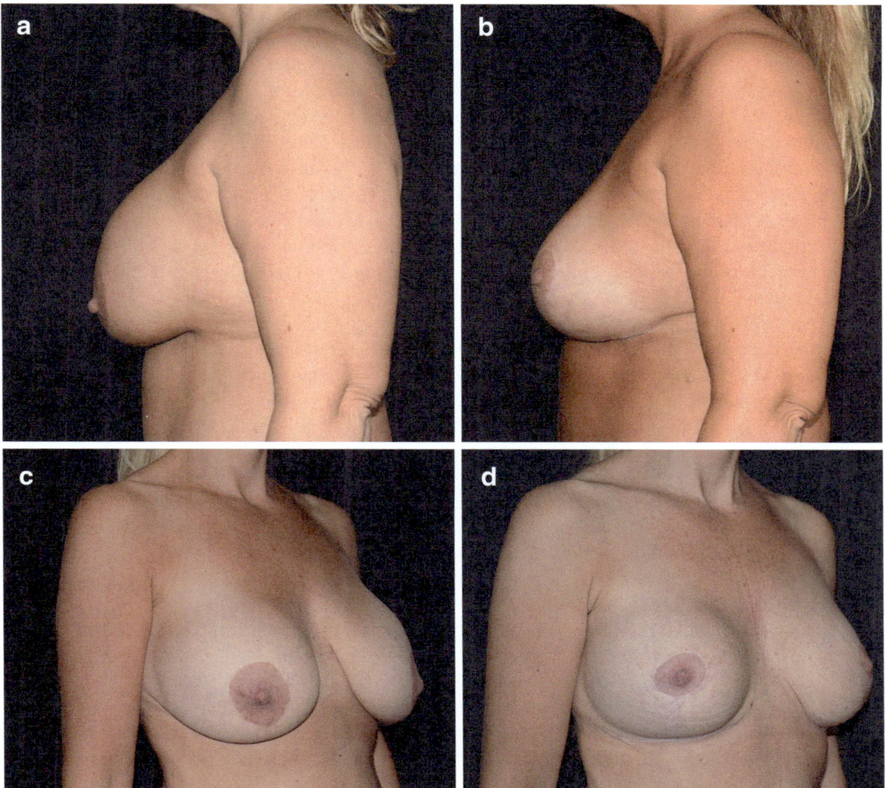

Fig. 10 Waterfall deformity corrected with implant exchange combined with a primary mastopexy. (**a** and **b**) Before and 1 year after implant exchange and primary mastopexy. (**c** and **d**) Before and 1 year after implant exchange and secondary mastopexy

References

1. Sarwer DB, Whitaker LA. Psychology of plastic and reconstructive surgery: a systematic clinical review. Plast Reconstr Surg. 2011:128(3):827–8. author reply 828–9.
2. Loch-Wilkinson A, et al. Breast implant-associated anaplastic large cell lymphoma in Australia and New Zealand: high-surface-area textured implants are associated with increased risk. Plast Reconstr Surg. 2017;140(4):645–54.
3. Castel N, Soon-Sutton T, Deptula P, Flaherty A, Don Parsa F. Polyurethane-coated breast implants revisited: a 30-year follow-up. Arch Plast Surg. 2015;42(2):186–93.
4. Barr S, Hill EW, Bayat AJ. Functional biocompatibility testing of silicone breast implants and a novel classification system based on surface roughness. Mech Behav Biomed Mate. 2017;75:75–81.
5. Jones P, Mempin M, Hu H, Chowdhury D, Foley M, Cooter R, Adams WP Jr, Vickery K, Deva AK. The functional influence of breast implant outer shell morphology on bacterial attachment and growth. Plast Reconstr Surg. 2018;142(4):837–49.

6. Atlan M, Nuti G, Wang H, Decker S, Perry T. Breast implant surface texture impacts hos tissue response. J Mech Behav Biomed Mater. 2018;88:377–85.
7. Wixtrom RN, Garadi V, Leopold J, Canady JW. Device-specific findings of imprinted texture breast implants: characteristics, risks, and benefits. Aesthet Surg J. 2020;40(2):167–73.
8. Hakelius L, Ohlsén L. Tendency to capsular contracture around smooth and textured silicone mammary implants: a five year follow up. Plast Reconstr Surg. 1997;100(6):1566–9.
9. Hammond DC, Canady JW, Love TR, Wixtrom RN, Caplin DA. Mentor contour profile gel implants: clinical outcomes at 10 years. Plast Reconstr Surg. 2017;140(6):1142–50.
10. Danino A, Rocher F, Blanchet-Bardorn C, Revol M, Servant JM. [A scanning electron microscopy study of the surface of porous-textured breast implants and their capsules. Description of the "velcro" effect of porous-textured breast prostheses]. Ann Chir Plast Esthet. 2001;46(1):23–30.
11. Al-Ajam Y, Marsh D, Mohan AT, Hamilton S. Assessing the augmented breast: a blinded study comparing round and anatomical form-stable implants. Aesthet Surg J. 2015;35(3):273–8.
12. Hidalgo DA, Weinstein AL. Intraoperative comparison of anatomical versus round implants in breast augmentation. Plast Reconstr Surg. 2017;139(3):587–96.
13. Friedman T, Davidovitch N, Scheflan M. Comparative double blind clinical study on round versus shaped cohesive gel implants. Aesthet Surg J. 2006;26(5):530–6.
14. Montemurro P, Adams WP Jr, Mallucci P, De Vita R, Layt C, Calobrace MB, Brown MH, Nava MB, Teitelbaum S, Del Yerro JLM, Bengtson B, Maxwell GP, Hedén P. Why do we need anatomical implants? The science and rationale for maintaining their availability and use in breast surgery. Aesthet Plast Surg. 2020;44(2):253–63.
15. Hedén P, Jernbeck J, Hober M. Breast augmentation with anatomical cohesive gel implants: the world's largest current experience. Clin Plast Surg. 2001;28(3):531–52.
16. Montemurro P, Papas A, Hedén P. Is rotation a concern with anatomical breast implants? A statistical analysis of factors predisposing to rotation. Plast Reconstr Surg. 2017;139(6):1367–78.
17. Sieber DA, Stark RY, Chase S, Schafer M, Adams WP. Clinical evaluation of shaped gel breast implant rotation using high-resolution ultrasound. Aesthet Surg J. 2017;37(3):290–6.
18. Adams WP Jr, Culbertson EJ, Deva AK, Magnusson MR, Layt C, Jewell ML, Mallucci P, Hedén P. Macrotextured breast implants with defined steps to minimize bacterial contamination around the device: experience in 42000 implants. Plast Reconstr Surg. 2017;140(3):427–31.
19. Maxwell GP, Birchenough SA, Gabriel A. Efficacy of neopectoral pocket in revisionary breast surgery. Aesthet Surg J. 2009;29(5):379–85. https://doi.org/10.1016/j.asj.2009.08.012.
20. Mallucci P, Branford OA. Concepts in aesthetic breast dimensions: analysis of the ideal breast. J Plast Reconstr Aesthet Surg. 2012;65(1):8–16.
21. Hedén P. Chapter 96. Breast augmentation with anatomical, high-cohesive silicon gel implants. In: Spear SL, editor. Surgery of the breast—principles and art, vol 2, Sect. 4. Philadelphia: Wolters Kluwer/Lippincott Williams & Wilkins. 2006. pp. 1344–1366.
22. Hedén P. Chapter 24. Form stable shaped high cohesive gel implants. In: Hall-Findlay EJ, Evans GRD, editors. Aesthtetic and reconstructive surgery of the breast. Philadelphia: Saunders Elsevier; 2010. p. 357–86.
23. Hedén P. Breast augmentation with anatomic, high-cohesiveness silicone gel implants (European experience). In: Spear SL, editor. Surgery of the breast: principles and art. 3rd ed. Philadelphia: Wolters Kluwer/Lippincott Williams & Wilkins; 2011. p. 1322–45.
24. Hedén P. Tissue based implant selection and preoperative markings with the AK or Q2 method. Aesthet Plast Surg. 2020;44(1):24–7. https://doi.org/10.1007/s00266-019-01534-y. Epub 2019 Nov 12. No abstract available.
25. Hedén P. Chapter 116. Shaped implants in breast augmentation. In: Gabriel A, Nahabedian M, Storm-Dickerson T, Maxwell GP, editors. Spear's surgery of the breast: principles and art. 4th ed. Philadelphia: Wolters Kluwer/Lippincott Williams & Wilkins; 2020.
26. Hedén P. Mastopexy augmentation with form stable breast implants. Clin Plast Surg. 2009;36(1):91–104.

Management of the Inframammary Fold

Maurizio Bruno Nava, Giuseppe Catanuto,
and Nicola Rocco

1 How to Reduce Complications and Malpositions with Accurate Preoperative Planning and Impeccable Surgical Technique

A scientific and rigorous approach towards breast augmentation is mandatory to reduce complication rates and to obtain high patient satisfaction level.

A rigorous approach starts with an accurate first consultation, analyzing the characteristics of the patient's skin and soft tissues, evaluating the size of the breast, the chest wall width and symmetry, assessing the breast shape and listening to patients' wishes, always remembering that if you fail to plan, you plan to fail.

After accurate planning and shared decision-making, a properly performed surgical procedure, with a complete knowledge of the devices you are using, and a correct and standardized follow-up are the other factors contributing to the best outcomes and the reduction of complications in breast augmentation.

Balancing the wishes of the patient with her tissue characteristics, identifying potential mismatches between the desired results and soft tissue characteristics are the first steps towards a successful breast augmentation. We must keep in mind that some choices in breast augmentation are not negotiable: the incision must always be preferred at the inframammary fold, chest width and cleavage will determine the choice of implant maximum width, the need of mastopexy could be not overcome with a larger volume implant. When the patient's wishes are not achievable, further consultation and patient education are mandatory. The more clearly the patient's

M. B. Nava (✉) · N. Rocco
G.Re.T.A. Group for Reconstructive and Therapeutic Advancements, Milan, Italy

G. Catanuto
G.Re.T.A. Group for Reconstructive and Therapeutic Advancements, Milan, Italy

Multidisciplinary Breast Unit, Azienda Ospedaliera Cannizzaro, Catania, Italy

© Springer Nature Switzerland AG 2022
R. de Vita (ed.), *Aesthetic Breast Augmentation Revision Surgery*,
https://doi.org/10.1007/978-3-030-86793-5_5

expectations are defined and the better her wishes are communicated, the more likely our goals can be achieved.

The final breast shape will depend on the characteristics of the coverage tissue (breast skin, glandular parenchyma and fat) and implants. Only after an objective assessment of specific patients' parameters (chest wall width, base width of the existing breast, nipple-to-inframammary fold distance under maximal gentle stretch, medial, lateral, superior, and central pinch thickness of the existing tissue, cleavage, and sternal notch to nipple distance) (Fig. 1), the surgeon can choose the best width, height, and projection of the implant.

We developed a planning method to guide the decisional process in breast augmentation based on skin and soft tissue characteristics, breast and chest wall size, breast shape and patient's wishes.

When planning a breast augmentation, the surgeon will assess implant size, implant type, implant pocket position, and incision location and each decision will strongly impact on final outcomes.

We must pursue evidence-based surgery, and to achieve predictable outcomes with low re-operation rates, we have to build our results on objective data.

Our decisional process in breast augmentation is summarized in the breast augmentation flow diagram (Fig. 2).

Potential surgical complications in breast implant surgery could be classified in preoperative and intraoperative complications and early and late postoperative complications (Fig. 3).

Preoperative complications essentially derive from poor planning (wrong choice of the surgical access, inaccurate measurements); intraoperative complications are associated to poor surgical technique. Early and late postoperative complications derive from all steps and even from poor management following the surgical procedure.

According to this classification, accurate preoperative planning could be viewed as the first step to reduce inframammary fold (IMF) violations.

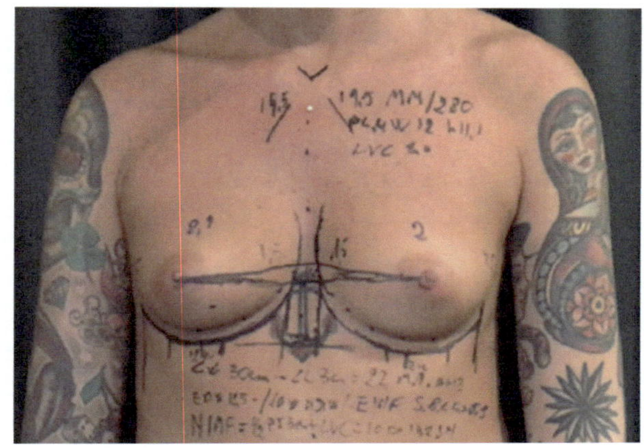

Fig. 1 Preoperative planning of breast augmentation. Key measurements: existing inframammary fold (e-IMF); new inframammary fold (N-IMF); breast parenchymal thickness; existing chest width; existing breast width; cleavage; lateral and medial pinch thickness; sternal notch to nipple distance (SN-N)

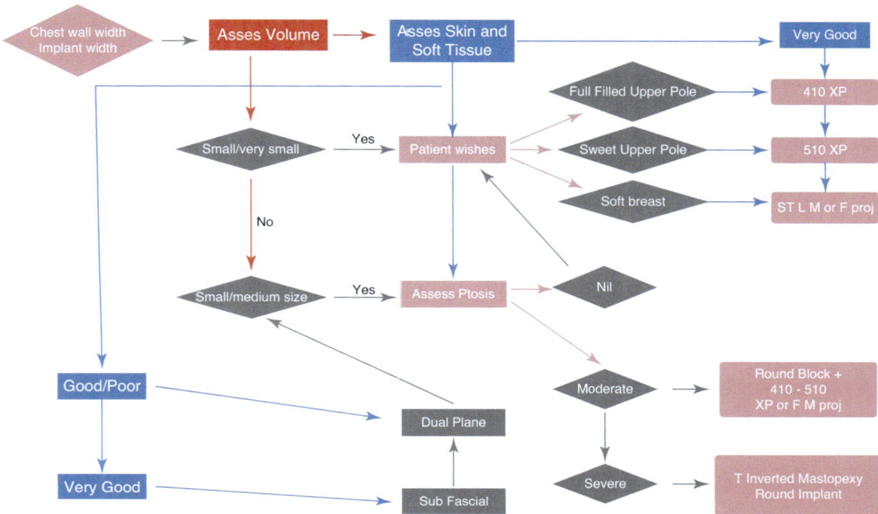

Fig. 2 The breast augmentation flow diagram

Pre- and intra-operative complications	Early post-operative complications	Late post-operative complications

• Poor planning
  - Incision
  - Incorrect measurement
• Bleeding
  - Surgical
  - Medical
• Over-dissection
• Implant malposition
• Pain
	• Haematoma
	• Seroma
	• Infection
	• Implant malposition
	• Pain
	• Implant Rupture
		• Infection
		• Seroma
		• Capsular contracture
		• Poor muscular animation (excessive, unusual, painful, distortion)
		• Implant visibility
		• Implant malposition (descent, double bubble, waterfall, etc)
		• Implant rippling and palpability
		• Synmastia
		• Poor scar healing, hypertrophy
		• Implant Rupture

Fig. 3 Authors' classification of complications

Inaccurate measurements or wrong position of the surgical access location could lead to the infringement of the IMF.

The first mistake that could be done when planning a breast augmentation is the wrong choice of implants: for instance, too big in relation to the patient's anatomical features, with the aim to fill a ptotic breast with redundant skin, instead of planning a mastopexy in association with the breast augmentation.

In order to avoid this potential mistake, we can suggest a useful tip when having the consultation with the patient. Ask the patient to lift up the hands as much as she can: if you cannot see the IMF, mastopexy is mandatory, not negotiable at all (Fig. 4). If we use an implant that is too big in order to fill the skin envelope (instead of correctly performing a mastopexy), we could easily experience early postoperative complications due to pain and tissue reactions that could lead to inflammation and capsular contracture, apart from clearly increasing the risk of breast ptosis and implant malposition, with breach of the IMF.

Another potential source of malpositions of the IMF is the wrong estimation of the level of the new IMF, where performing the surgical incision. We advice to strongly prefer IMF incisions to minimize contaminations and to perfectly recreate the new IMF position. During my planning this is not negotiable at all. I perfectly know that another choice could increase my complication rate. However the surgical access will be defined according to the patient's wishes and surgical skills trying to reduce tissue trauma and trade-offs. A peri-areolar access could be chosen if a peri-areolar scar is already present and the patient desire not to have other scars. Anyway in case of peri-areolar access, the gland must not be passed through, only small volume implants could be used and the patient must be informed about the higher risk of complications and IMF malpositions.

Several methods have been described in order to define the level of the new IMF, as the ICE principle [1], the method reported by Tebbetts with the TEPID system [2] or that described by Heden et al. [3]. We prefer to calculate the position of the new IMF (distance between the nipple and the new IMF) adding the half parenchymal pinch thickness to the implant's Lower Ventral Curvature (LVC). It is important to mark the new IMF position on full gentle stretch of the skin and

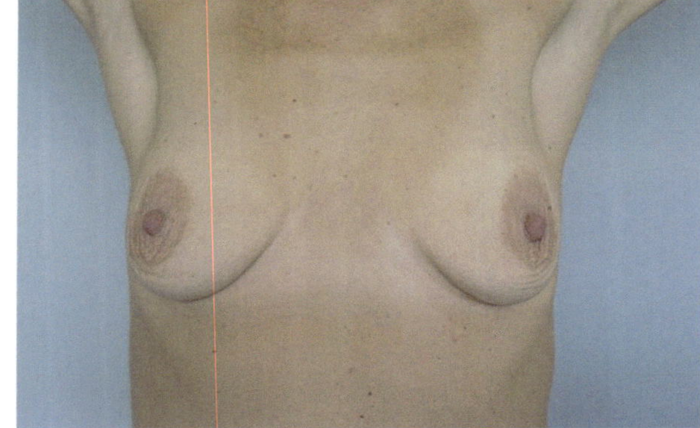

Fig. 4 How to choose if needing a mastopexy or not in association with a breast augmentation. Ask the patient to lift up the hands over her head as much as she can: if you cannot see the inframammary fold, a mastopexy is mandatory, as in this case

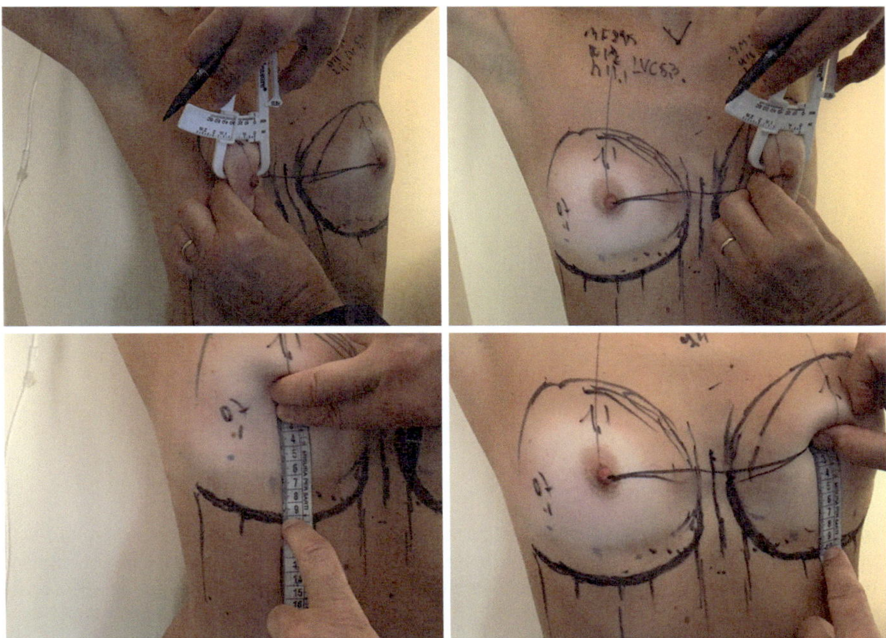

Fig. 5 Authors' method to define the level of the new IMF. We calculate the position of the new IMF (distance between the nipple and the new IMF) adding the half parenchymal thickness to the implant's lower ventral curvature (LVC). It is important to mark the new IMF position on full gentle stretch of the skin and patients' hands on the head

patients hands on the head (Fig. 5). We prefer to use the half pinch thickness plus the LVC better than the half implant height and LVC as described by Mallucci and Heden [1, 3], as the maximum implant projection for anatomical implants with different projection and same width is in the same position (Fig. 6), thus basing the estimations of the new IMF location on the height of the implant could lead to suboptimal results.

Complications and malpositions could also derive from intraoperative mistakes.

In order to reduce malpositions of the IMF, it is of primary relevance to properly close the IMF when using an inframammary approach. It is important to fix the IMF on the pectoralis major, pinching the muscle with the stitch that will close the fascia superficialis at the IMF (Fig. 7). Note that both in a subglandular and in a dual plane approach it will be possible to fix the stitches to the pectoralis major as also in a dual plane approach a strip of muscle will be left on the thoracic wall when the pectoralis major is cut at different levels according to Tebbetts' classification [4].

Following this rigorous approach towards breast augmentation, the rates of malpositions of the IMF will be significantly reduced, but if a malposition in the IMF would occur, the surgeon should know how to properly manage and solve it.

The chance of managing IMF position defects starts with an accurate knowledge of the characteristics and anatomy of this area.

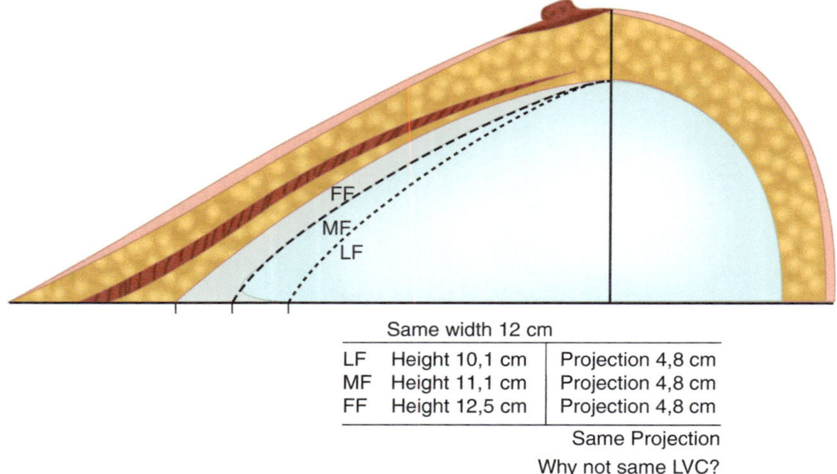

Fig. 6 Defining the position of the new IMF. Author's personal drawings. We prefer to use the half pinch thickness plus the LVC better than the half implant height and LVC, as the maximum implant projection for anatomical implants with different projection and same width is in the same position, thus basing the estimations of the new IMF location on the height of the implant could lead to suboptimal results

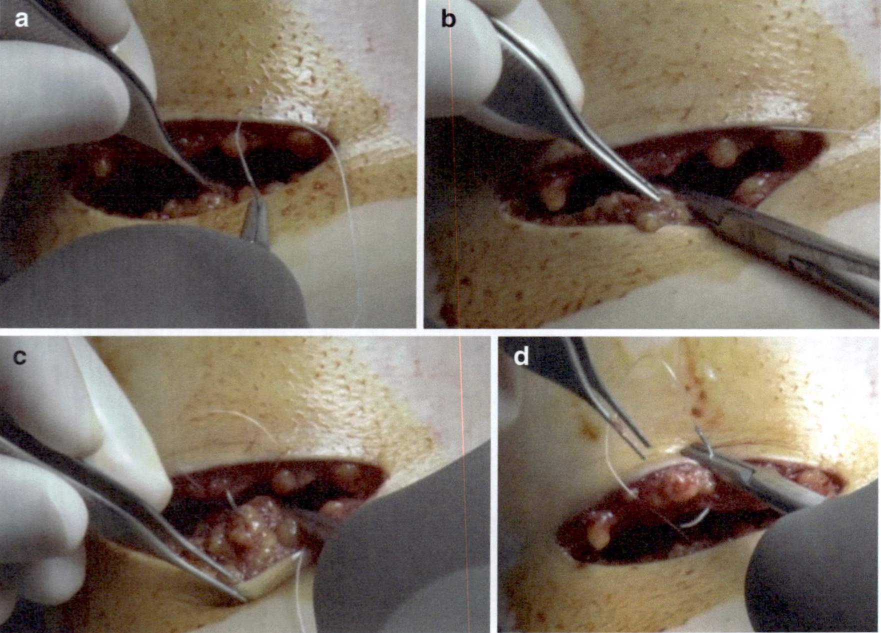

Fig. 7 Closure of the inframammary access. (**a**) Pinch the pectorals major; (**b**) Pass the stitch through the pectorals major fibers first; (**c**) Pass the same stitch through the inferior edge of the fascia superficialis; (**d**) Pass the stitch on the superior edge of the fascia superficialis and close it in an inverting fashion; (**e**) Final result

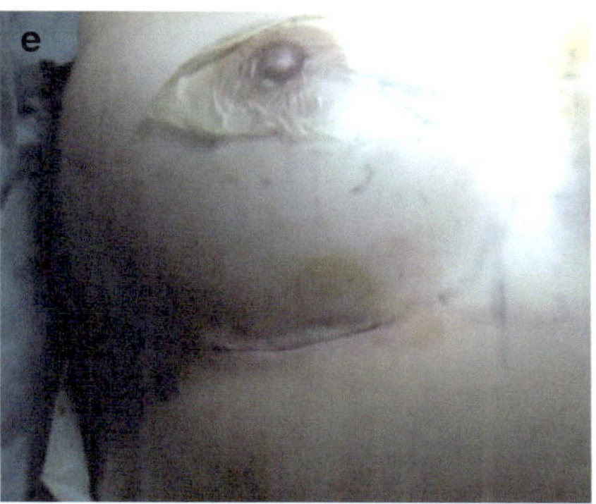

Fig. 7 (continued)

2   The Inframammary Fold

The inframammary fold represents one of the primary elements in breast aesthetics. The harmony of the breast is related to four IMF characteristics: contour, level, angle, and symmetry.

Contour represents the lower base of the breast on the thoracic wall, appearing as an uninterrupted visual line composed of three parts: the midpoint (i.e., the lowest point of the fold) and two segments, medial and lateral, respectively. The course draws a convex arch downward as being C-shaped, U-shaped, or nearly horizontal.

Level is at the fifth and sixth ribs, with the lowest part usually reaching the sixth intercostal space. The average distance from the areola is 5.5–7 cm for small breasts and 7–9 or more cm for large breasts. This transverse level is usually proportioned to the chest width and patient's height. The proportion of the upper breast pole to the lower pole is a 45:55 ratio, the angulation of the nipple is upwards at a mean angle of 20° from the nipple meridian, the upper pole slope is linear or slightly concave and the lower pole is convex [5].

Angle derives from the intersection of the lower profile of the breast with the thoracic plane. It is related to breast ptosis. An open angle appears in small nonptotic breasts. A 90-degree or something more angle accentuates the beauty of a youthful breast. In contrast, a sharp angle that appears in large breasts, also having a fascial laxity, is typical of elderly breasts and can be less pleasant. The IMF angle is one of the most important features in the aesthetic appearance of the breast.

Symmetry depends on the previous characteristics as comparing the left with the right side. Breast harmony largely depends on symmetry and embraces two kinds of symmetry: metric and visual. Metric symmetry must be of concern during the preoperative approach but surgeons should always be aware of the patient's wishes and body self-perception that are related to visual symmetry rather than to metric symmetry.

Anatomical landmarks are fundamental in creating IMF contour and level and the angle sharpness, due to breast ptosis and weight, is deeply influenced by the modifications of the fascial system by aging. A clarification of the IMF anatomic structure is needed to understand the unique nature of IMF as a separate anatomic unit and for recreating it when the patient experiences the bad results of a previous breast augmentation, with a malposition of the IMF (asymmetry, bottoming out, double bubble deformity, etc.).

3   Anatomy of the Inframammary Fold

There are three anatomic aspects of the superficial fascia that produce the IMF with no reference to large-scale structures as ligaments.

First, IMF appears to be a zone of subcutaneous adherence (thick retinacula between the superficial and deep fascia), where contiguous connective structures of both superficial and deep subcutaneous layers persist as different anatomic micro units of the same fascial frame, according to the concept of the skin-superficial/fat-superficial fascial system functional unit described by Lockwood [6] and applied in the study published by Nava et al. [7].

Second, the superficial fascia of the inframammary region, direct prolongation of the abdominal one, extends to the retromammary space above the deep (muscular) fascia, deepening the level where IMF starts. The deeper plane is generated by the changing thickness of the deep subcutaneous layer that, in the abdomen, is separated from the deep fascia by a fatty layer, whereas, in the submammary region, this layer becomes more fibrous than fatty and hence thinner. The sternal depression, similarly due to absence of fat in the deep layer and presence of adherent retinacula, can become a true fold in obese people.

Third, the superficial fascial layer is a constant fibrous membrane thicker in the inframammary zone and in the whole abdomen (also called Scarpa's), than in the retromammary zone of the female breast. Its thickening increases in time due to the action of breast weight.

Another important issue to clarify is how to merge the inframammary frame of the superficial fascial system with the entire connective frame of the mammary gland.

The Cooper's ligaments detach from the superficial fascia and go up to the skin. The same behavior can be observed regarding the capsular envelope, which is a fascial annex covering the anterior surface of the mammary gland. Such a fibrous band is made of merging thick retinacula, more apparent at IMF, at the site of detachment from the superficial fascia. This is the fibrous membrane that many authors confuse with the inframammary ligament: it can be interconnected to the muscular fascia through the superficial fascia; it can be joined to the presternal fascia at the medial extremity; the orientation follows the breast shape instead of the pectoral inferior border; the density and thickness are related to age, breast size, and weight. It is not a true ligament but rather the capsule of a gland of ectodermal origin.

It is important to underline that the IMF anatomy has been debated for many decades and it is strictly linked to the theories about the two-layered [8–11] or uni-layered [12–14] superficial fascia. The fold had always been neglected by anatomists, perhaps because they did not believe it to have anatomic identity, even though it would appear to have a constant position.

Based on the authors' anatomic dissections on fresh cadavers, histologic and surgical investigations conducted on live dissections [7, 15], it can be asserted that there is not a macrostructure featuring the IMF, but that its anatomic fundamentals lay on a special microstructure as totally generated by the superficial fascial system.

A clear and correct understanding of the anatomy will facilitate surgeons in safe-guarding the IMF and rebuilding the interrupted frame after breast augmentation and IMF malposition.

4   How to Recreate the Inframammary Fold by Means of the Superficial Fascial System Following Malpositioning Subsequent to Breast Augmentation

Dealing with malpositioning of the inframammary fold following breast augmentation is a challenging task. We will try to offer some useful tips to correct different types of inframammary fold malpositioning.

A correct planning allows surgeons to decide how to reshape the inferior pole of the breast, the level of ptosis, and the IMF positioning to correct a bottoming out or a double bubble deformity.

The surgeon could face two possible IMF malpositions: the IMF could be in higher or lower position compared to that of an ideal breast, due to poor planning, wrong choice of the implant, or inaccurate surgical technique.

Preoperatively the IMF level is marked as being equal to the contralateral one. Preoperative planning is of primary importance in order to reach a good cosmetic result as for each breast surgical procedure.

First, it is important to identify the inframammary fold level. The second step will be the identification of the existing skin incision, discussing with the patient the possibility of a new one. We advice to use an IMF approach that could be on the previous surgical access or a new incision, being the previous completely dislocated or peri-areolar only if a peri-areolar scar is already present, the patient refuses other scars even though informed of higher risk of complications and always without passing through the gland, to reduce contamination.

If the patient refuses other scars apart from the previous peri-areolar one, even though well informed about the possibility of higher complication rates, you can follow the subsequent step to improve the IMF location and definition.

If the implant is dislocated upward, the dissection must reach the IMF level; in contrast, when the implant is displaced downward, the lower skin envelope must be lifted up and then fixed at the new level. When feasible, we prefer to perform a total capsulectomy or, if possible, to preserve a portion of the capsule to better define the IMF. If this is not possible, both scoring and resection of the capsular and scar tissue of the lower pole of the breast are the first maneuvers to expand the implant pocket and to expose the deep subcutaneous layer.

The IMF incision will release the superficial fascia along the new IMF contour. Then the lower of the two newly scored edges is grasped, this action dragging the superficial fascial system upward with a smooth and easy effect on the skin. This is the right position where the sutures to recreate the IMF should be positioned. The thoracic anchorage is safely given by the fibrous capsular tissue created around the previous implant. The fold is recreated pinching the posterior aspect of the capsule on the pectorals major muscle (if following a subglandular or dual plane approach) or on the thoracic wall (if following a submuscular approach), then passing the same stitch through the inferior edge of the fascia superficialis, so on the superior edge of the fascia superficialis and closing it in an inverting fashion.

The suture will fix the fascia superficialis to the thoracic wall (if following a previous sub pectoral approach) or to the pectorals major (if following a sub glandular or dual plane approach). It is important to externally check the right placement step by step, always using the seated position for the patient, the supine position modifying the IMF level.

We present some examples of different malpositions of the IMF, analyzing the causes leading to the poor outcome and the best technique to properly and effectively correct them (Figs. 8, 9, 10, and 12).

In Fig. 8 we present a case of IMF asymmetry due to poor planning, wrong choice of the implant and surgical technique with a totally submuscular implant positioning (A). The chosen peri-areolar access contributed to the poor result and to

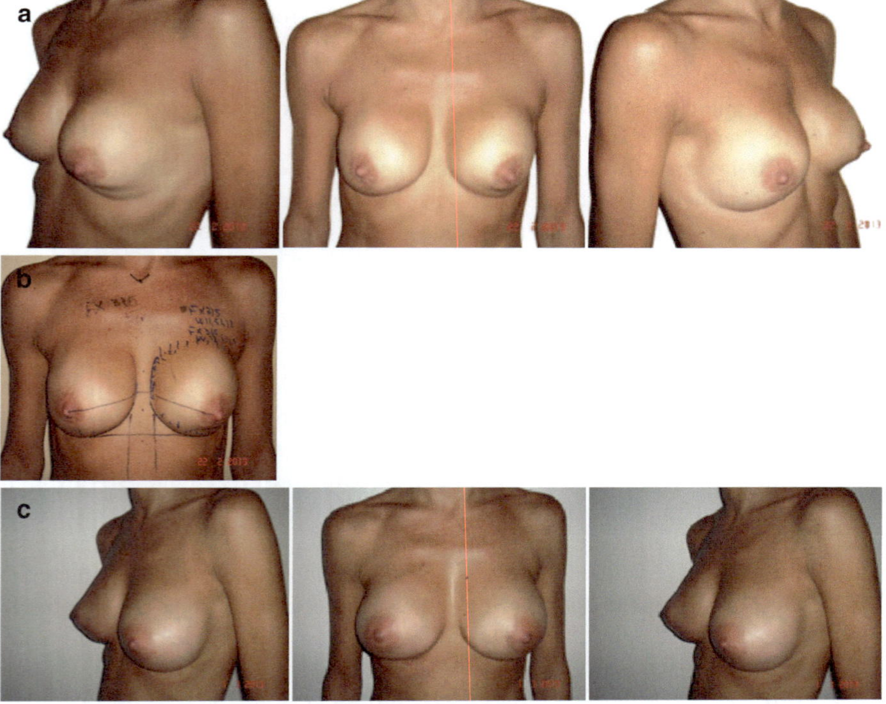

Fig. 8 (**a**) Inframammary fold asymmetry and capsular contracture. (**b**) Preoperative markings; (**c**) Correction with a dual plane approach with anatomical implants

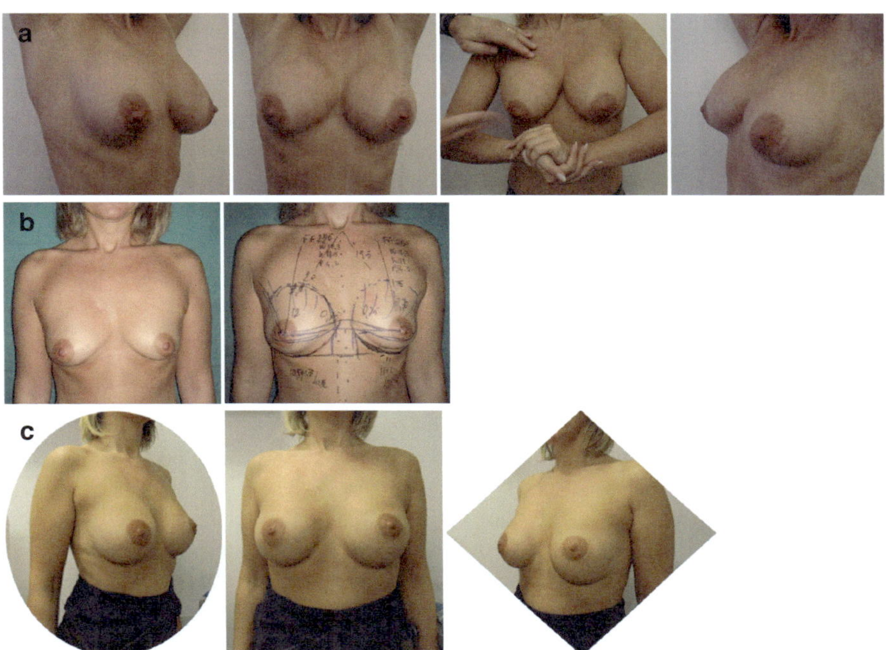

Fig. 9 (**a**) Inframammary fold asymmetry and synmastia. (**b**) Two-stage corrective approach. Removal of the implants and re-operation at 6 months (preoperative markings); (**c**) Secondary breast augmentation; postoperative results

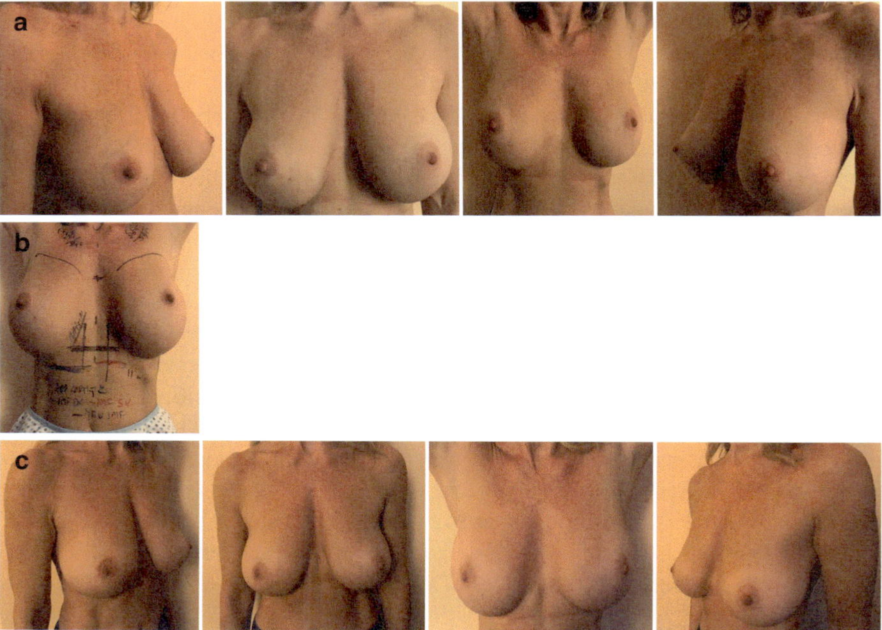

Fig. 10 (**a**) Inframammary fold asymmetry. (**b**) Preoperative markings. (**c**) Postoperative results

the capsular contracture development. According to patient's wishes, we opted to correct the poor outcome using an anatomical implant, a new IMF surgical access (see preoperative drawings in box B). After incising the skin and the fascia superficialis, we reached the pectorals major muscle and created a dual plane. We performed a total dome capsulectomy and partial capsulectomy on the chest wall, pro-active hemostasis and selective releasing of the medial pectoralis major fibers with the aim of reducing animation deformities. Then we defined and sutured the IMF as shown in Fig. 7.

In Fig. 9 we show a case of IMF asymmetry and synmastia (A). In this case the poor aesthetic result and asymmetry between the IMFs are related to a poor preoperative planning (too big pre-pectoral round implants) and a poor surgical technique with the creation of too large implant pockets and implant malposition. We considered a two-stage corrective approach, after thorough patient information, in order to reach an optimal outcome. We removed the implants, performed a total capsulectomy and re-operation at 6 months (see preoperative markings in box B); in box C we show the postoperative results of the secondary breast augmentation with peri-areolar approach, anatomical implant positioning, total detachment of the gland from the fascia superficialis to reach the muscle without passing through the gland and dual plane technique. The IMF has been defined as described above, in the case we have to use a pre-existing peri-areolar skin incision. When dealing with a synmastia, we advice to follow a two-stage approach, removing the implants and delaying re-intervention after at least 6 months, when planning the procedure as a primary augmentation. Treating those patients requires a significant patient engagement and a thorough patient information.

In Fig. 10 we show a case of IMF asymmetry due to poor planning, wrong choice of the implants (too big round implants), and poor surgical technique (subglandular implant positioning without a proper suture of the new IMF and sliding of the implant under the fascia superficialis). You can see both IMFs below the level of the surgical scars (A). We show preoperative markings in box B. We created a new implant pocket in a dual plane position (type 2 according to Tebbetts' classification) using pro-active hemostasis and selective releasing of medial pectoralis major muscle fibers, as usual. The new pocket has been created leaving the implant inside, in order to ease the surgical maneuvers and sparing a portion of the capsule to avoid pectoralis major retractions (Fig. 11). Anatomical implants have been used according to patient's wishes. We recreated the IMF using the same surgical access but correctly closing the different layers as described in Fig. 7.

In Fig. 12 we show a case of double bubble due to a serious planning mistake. A mastopexy would have been advisable in association with the first augmentation, as described above (Fig. 4). According to patient's wishes, we decided to avoid new scars and consequently a mastopexy has not been performed. The correction has been performed using the superficial fascia system and the same implants (anatomical implants). The result is still not perfect but the patient was satisfied and no other surgery has been performed (postoperative result at 25 years in box B).

If the lower pole is too thin, we advice to use ADMs or synthetic meshes, according to personal experience. Using an ADM means to use one more device, thus

Fig. 11 Tips to create a
new implant pocket. How
to create a new dual plane:
leave the capsule inside
when possible, to avoid
pectoralis major muscle
retractions

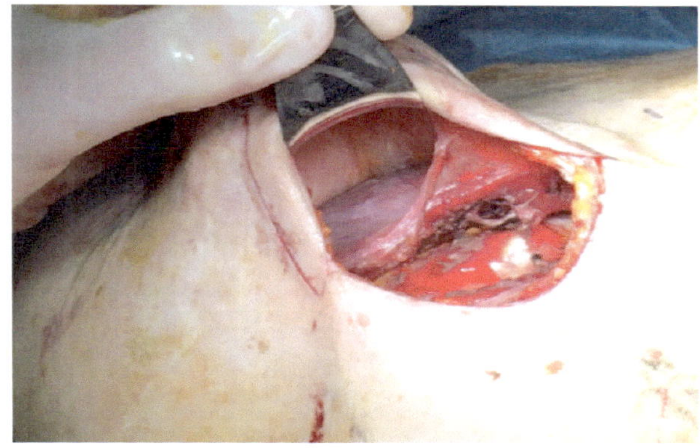

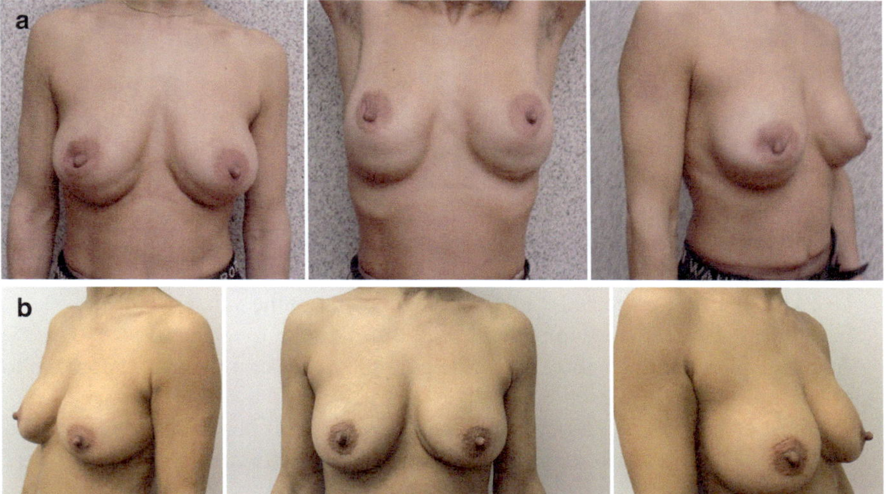

Fig. 12 (**a**) Double bubble. (**b**) Correction using the superficial fascia system and the same anatomical implant. Postoperative result at 25 years

increasing the risk of complications or side effects. We suggest to use ADMs or
synthetic meshes only if really needed. The ADMs must be sutured at the level of
the new IMF with the patient seated, as described above. I suggest to preoperatively
mark three lines where to fix the first three stitches and then to go ahead with a running suture from the medial inferior edge of the IMF to the inferior lateral one. I
suggest to use reabsorbable sutures. When a capsule is present and there are no
reasons to perform a capsulectomy, it is possible to spare an inferior pedicled capsular flap and to recreate the IMF using it as an ADM.

We could summarize some key consideration in revision breast surgery to correct
post-breast augmentation deformities (Fig. 13):

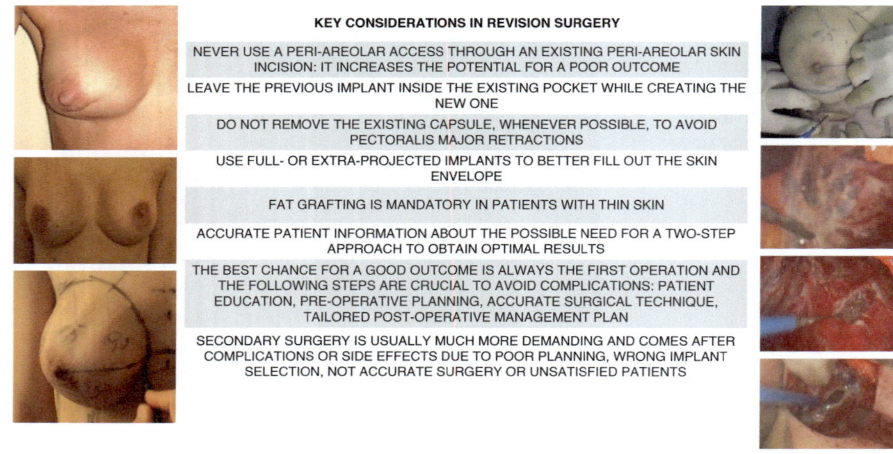

Fig. 13 Key considerations in revision surgery

- Never use a peri-areolar approach through an existing peri-areolar incision: it increases the potential for a poor outcome.
- Leave the previous implant inside the existing pocket while creating the new pocket.
- Do not remove the existing capsule, whenever possible, with the aim of avoiding pectoralis major retractions.
- Use Full or Extra-projected implants to better fill out the skin envelope.
- Fat grafting is mandatory in patients with thin skin.
- Accurate patient information about the possible need for a two-step approach to obtain optimal results.
- The best chance for a good outcome is always the first operation and the following steps are crucial to avoid complications: *patient education, preoperative planning, accurate surgical technique, tailored postoperative management plan.*
- Secondary surgery is usually much more demanding and comes after complications or side effects due to poor planning, wrong implant selection, not accurate surgery, or unsatisfied patients.

References

1. Mallucci P, Branford OA. Augmentation: the ICE principle. Design for natural breast. Plast Reconstr Surg. 2016;137(6):1728–37.
2. Tebbetts JB. A system for breast implant selection based on patient tissue characteristics and implant-soft tissue dynamics. Plast Reconstr Surg. 2002;109(4):1396–409.
3. Hedén P, Jernbeck J, Hober M. Breast augmentation with anatomical cohesive gel implants: the world's largest current experience. Clin Plast Surg. 2001;28(3):531–52.

4. Tebbetts JB. Dual plane breast augmentation: optimizing implant-soft-tissue relationships in a wide range of breast types. Plast Reconstr Surg. 2006;118(7 Suppl):81S–98S; discussion 99S–102S.
5. Mallucci P, Branford OA. Concepts in aesthetic breast dimensions: analysis of the ideal breast. J Plast Reconstr Aesthet Surg. 2012;65(1):8–16.
6. Lockwood TE. Superficial fascial system (SFS) of the trunk and extremities: a new concept. Plast Reconstr Surg. 1991;87:1009–18.
7. Nava M, Quattrone P, Riggio E. Focus on the breast fascial system: a new approach for inframammary fold reconstruction. Plast Reconstr Surg. 1998;102:1034–45.
8. Bostwick J III. Anatomy and physiology. In: Plastic and reconstructive breast surgery. St. Louis: Quality Medical; 1990. p. 67.
9. Rieffel H. L'appareil génital de la femme. In: Traité d'Anatomie Humaine Publié sur la Direction de P.Poirier et A.Charpy. T. 5, Fasc.I. Paris: Masson; 1901.
10. Chiarugi G. Istituzioni di Anatomia dell'Uomo. Milan; 1908.
11. Sterzi G. La fascia superficiale. In: Il tessuto sottocutaneo (tela subcutanea). Ricerche anatomiche. Firenze: L.Niccolai; 1910. pp. 62–8.
12. Bayati S, Seckel BR. Inframammary crease ligament. Plast Reconstr Surg. 1995;95:501–8.
13. Van Straalen WH, Hage JJ, Bloemena E. The inframammary ligament: myth or reality? Ann Plast Surg. 1995;35:237–41.
14. Garnier D, Antonin R, Foulon P, et al. Le sillon sous-mammaire: mythe ou réalité? Ann Chir Plast Esther. 1991;36:313–9.
15. Riggio E, Quattrone P, Nava M. Anatomical study of the breast superficial fascial system: the inframammary fold unit. Eur J Plast Surg. 2000;23:310–5.

Synmastia

Roy de Vita and Buccheri Ernesto Maria

1 Introduction

Synmastia is a rare serious congenital condition that is described as a connection between the breasts with or without macromastia; there is accumulation of fat and glandular tissue between the breasts, which produces a unified appearance of the breast tissue across the chest. Relatively more frequent is acquired synmastia that can occur after augmentation mammaplasty [1].

Although developmental synmastia can occur without surgery, this chapter will put attention only to synmastia correction after breast surgery with implant uses.

Synmastia after breast augmentation has been categorized as "crossing of the midline, even if it is only on one side"; "central webbing of the breasts"; "disruption of the midline sternal attachments"; "medial confluence of the breasts"; and "displacement of one or both implants beyond the midline." This is previously described as moderate (bicapsular synmastia), when some muscle fibers and/or soft tissue connect the midsternal skin to the underlying sternum on one side or severe (monocapsular synmastia) when there is communication between the two periprosthetic capsules [1–8].

For our convenience we consider the definition of synmastia when the breast implant crosses the midline. A lot of surgical techniques for repair are described in literature [6]. As reported in the literature, iatrogenic acquired synmastia is characterized by any kind of previous breast implant positioning for aesthetic augmentation or reconstructive purposes [9].

R. de Vita
Department of Plastic Surgery, National Institute for Cancer, "Regina Elena", Rome, Italy

B. E. Maria (✉)
Medicinaplasticaroma Center, Plastic Surgery, Rome, Italy
e-mail: buccheri@medicinaplasticaroma.it

© Springer Nature Switzerland AG 2022
R. de Vita (ed.), *Aesthetic Breast Augmentation Revision Surgery*,
https://doi.org/10.1007/978-3-030-86793-5_6

We describe our surgical approach for synmastia correction that consist in implant removal, capsulectomy, pectoralis major muscle repositioning, change the plane from subpectoral to prepectoral positioning, and subdermal-perichondral stiches to maintain and reinforce the parasternal medial line bilaterally.

Our described technique is fast, simple, and reproducible for reliable, stable, and firm long last results.

2 Preoperative Evaluation and Planning

The first essential step to a correct planning of the synmastia correction procedure is a preoperative consultation conducted by the plastic surgeon combined with the patients' clinical exams. The anamestic data are recorded and the patient is investigated about her previous breast surgeries including information about breast implant brand and size; other general information are requested such as health status, smoking habits, pregnancies and lactations, and weight history including fluctuation, major changes, and surgical weight loss. Breast health evaluation should include past history of breast cancer, abnormal mammograms, as well as a summary of previous surgeries, if any. Surgeon should also ask the patient for self-awareness of any pre-existing breast asymmetry and assess asymmetry grade by clinical exam and preoperative photo-documentation. All these assessments will help in achieving the desired aesthetic goals and avoiding patient's dissatisfaction [10].

Preoperative markings on the skin are made with the patient in the standup position. Firstly, the surgeon should outline the new standard breast landmarks: sternal notch, chest midline from sternal notch to xyphoid apophysis, breast lateral-lines, and infra-mammary folds (IMF). Moreover it is important to mark the parasternal vertical midlines at 1.5–2 cm parallel to the chest midline according with the emitorax width also considering the right positioning of the new breast mound. We always use the previous scar to avoid any additional one. Implant volume is determined for each patient in accordance with the desired cup size and the breast/thoracic measurements (width and height of breast base, thoracic circumference, jugular-to-nipple distance, nipple-to-nipple distance, and nipple-to-IMF distance). When pinching test is less than 2 cm we use the prepectoral approach in any way performing hybrid breast augmentation, so we use autologous fat graft to improve implant tissue coverage as well described before in Literature.

3 Surgical Technique

Procedure is performed under general anesthesia, with the patient in a semi-seated position and abducted arms. We recommend the following sequence for optimal repair. The skin incision is conducted by retracing the previous scar. First, capsulectomy is performed trying to remove implant and capsule integrally. If the pectoralis major muscle is relatively close to the sternum, is preferable repositioning and repair it from posteriorly to the more medial and inferior position as possible, we recommend 2/0 polyglactin 910 (Vicryl, Ethicon J&J sutures) as a running suture. At this point, we feel strongly that placing another implant under the muscle will likely condemn the patient to the same problem in the future. Many patients came to us after multiple attempts at repair returning the implants to the retromuscular position. So we always prefer to change the plane and place the new implant under the gland in a prepectoral positioning.

Previous implant sizers uses we choose the definitive smaller one, anatomical or round, according with preop pinching test, emithorax width and height and patient cup desires as well described in our previous studies [10]. At this time of the surgery we always prefer to reinforce the new pocket with single subdermal to periosteum 2/0 polyglactin 910 (Vicry, Ethicon J&J sutures) single stiches avoiding any possibilities of revisional surgery. The single stitches are located at the parasternal level 1.5–2 cm laterally and bilaterally to the midline and, according to the needs, will be one up to three for each side; the evident pinching cutaneous effect in the immediate postop period will disappear in 3–6 months leaving a pleasant and effective long last result. When pinching test is less than 2 cm we use the prepectoral approach any way performing hybrid breast augmentation, so autologous fat graft is used to improve implant tissue coverage as well described before in Literature [10, 11].

4   Postoperative Care

A compression dressing with gauze and cotton is applied immediately after the surgery. Then, within 24 h postoperatively, the dressing is replaced with a sports bra which the patients are advised to continue wearing for 6 weeks. Patient is discharged with a prescription for oral analgesics and a full course of oral antibiotic prophylaxis after 1 or 2 nights of hospital stay. Drains are left in place until the first follow-up visit, usually scheduled 3–5 days after the surgery. Antibiotic prophylaxis is discontinued after the drain removal at the first follow-up visit if the amount of fluid collected is <50 mL within the 24 h. Further follow-up visits and photograph are scheduled at 1, 3, 6 months, and 1 year postoperatively. A complete case is reported as shown in Figs. 1, 2, 3, 4, 5, 6, 7. 8, and 9.

5   Discussion

Synmastia was first described in 1983 as the medial confluence of the breast mounds. It exists in 2 forms: congenital and iatrogenic. Although literature is present regarding congenital synmastia, with the rise in breast augmentation over the past few decades, the mechanisms by which iatrogenic synmastia appears have been investigated more thoroughly. 2 Iatrogenic (or acquired) synmastia after breast augmentation has been attributed to displacement of implants over the sternum, disruption of midline sternal fascia, and over-dissection of the medial major pectoralis muscle attachments to the sternum [1, 3–5].

Fig. 1 Preoperative synmastia frontal view, 32-year-old nulliparous woman after 1 year subpectoral breast augmentation with 375 round texturized implant

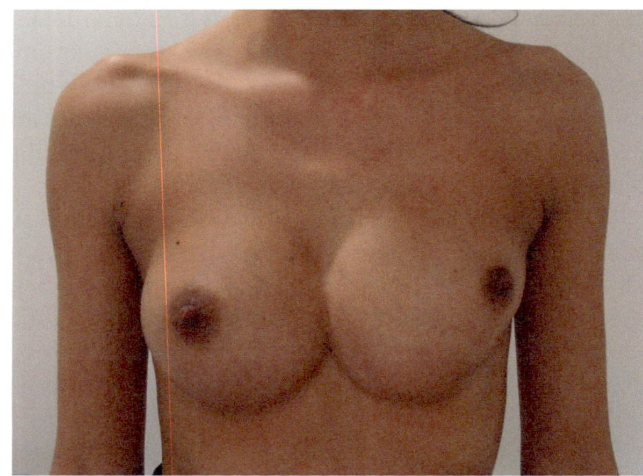

Fig. 2 Postoperative 14 days frontal view after subglandular synmastia correction by using 300 cc texturized anatomical implant, the single subdermal to periosteum 2/0 polyglactin 910 (Vicry, Ethicon J&J sutures) stiches are still visible

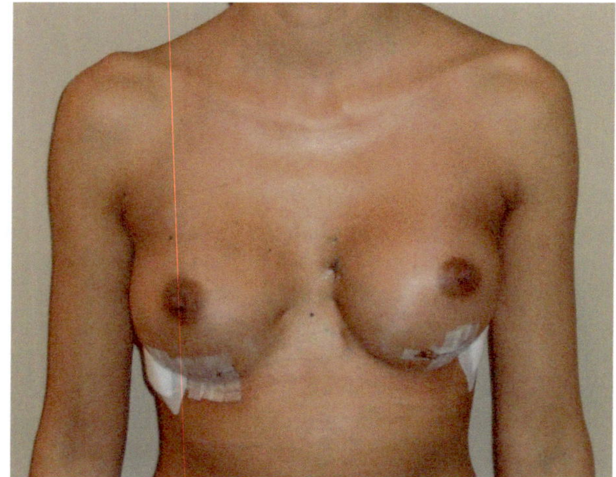

Fig. 3 Postoperative 12 months frontal view

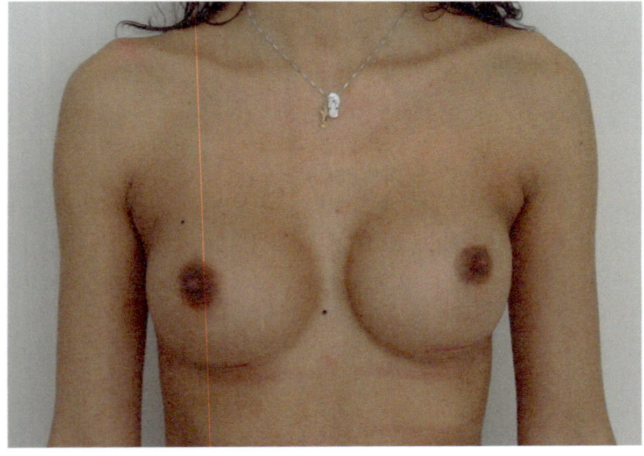

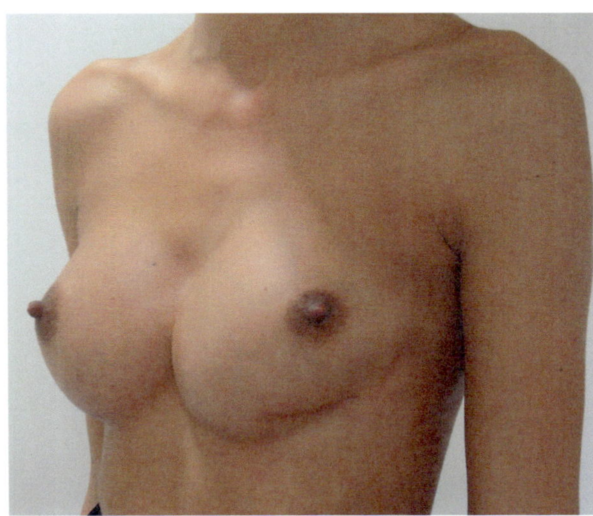

Fig. 4 Preoperative three quarter left view

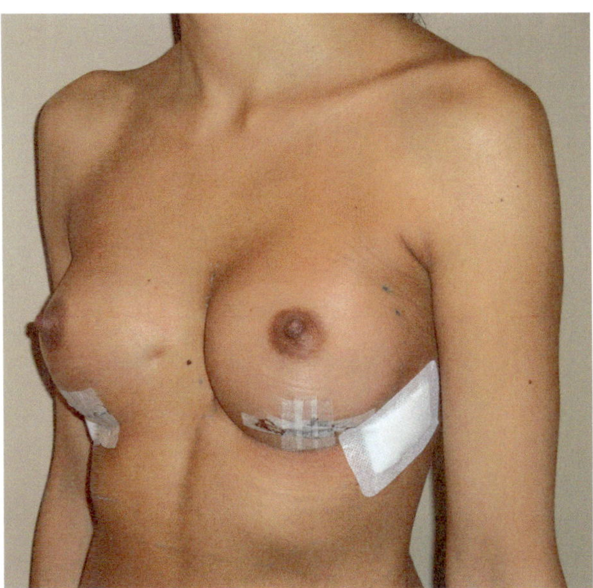

Fig. 5 Postoperative 14 days three quarter left view

Based on our experience and literature review, postaugmentation synmastia is present with high range of patients that had undergone more than one breast surgery and the majority of them had undergone secondary surgeries to augment the breast size; many of them had large implants, arbitrarily defined by us as greater than 450 cc or with a diameter of 14 cm or more. Some of the patients had associated chest wall skeletal deformities, and some had undergone simultaneous mastopexy at the time of their breast enlargement. The last but not the least, postaugmentation

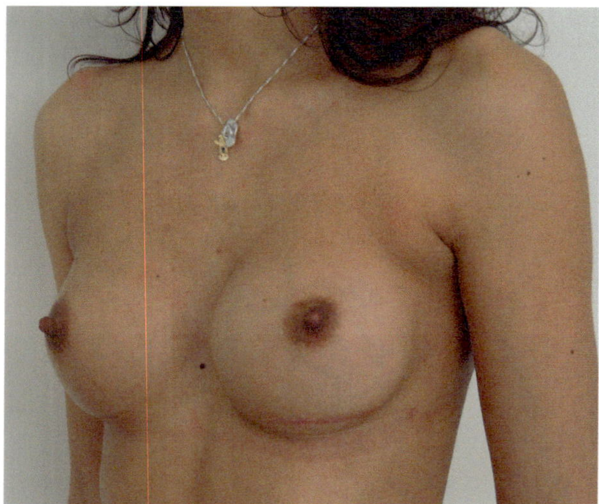

Fig. 6 Postoperative 12 months three quarter left view

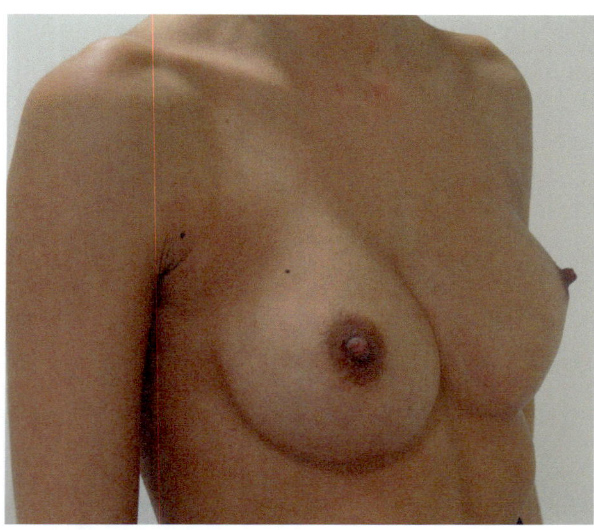

Fig. 7 Preoperative three quarter right view

synmastia is quite always reported when the implants were located in a subpectoral pocket [12]. Sanchez et al. showed in their anatomical dissections that in some cadavers the pectoralis major muscles can be as thin as 3–4 mm at the origin along the sternum from the second to fifth ribs [13, 14]. Kalaria et al. believe that patients who have this thin origin are at risk of tearing their sternal muscle origin of the pectoralis major muscle after subpectoral bilateral augmentation mammaplasty. In a previous cadaveric dissections study it is revealed that the pectoralis major and pectoralis minor muscles frequently have inconsistent origins from their costal attachments at the sternum. They declare that during subpectoral breast

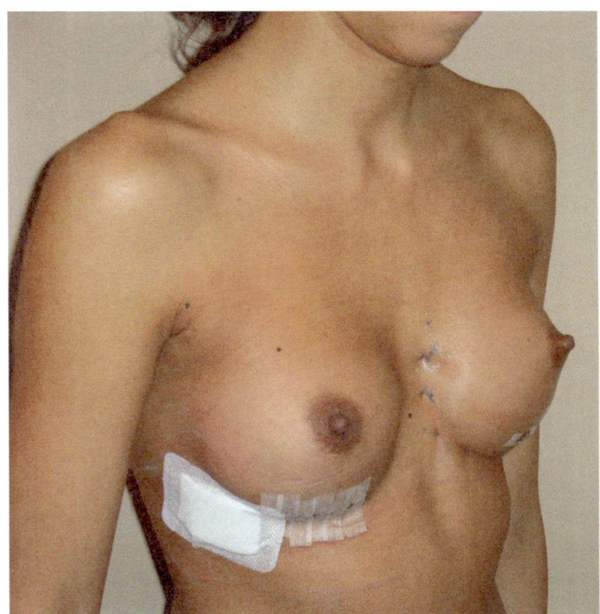

Fig. 8 Postoperative 14 days three quarter right view

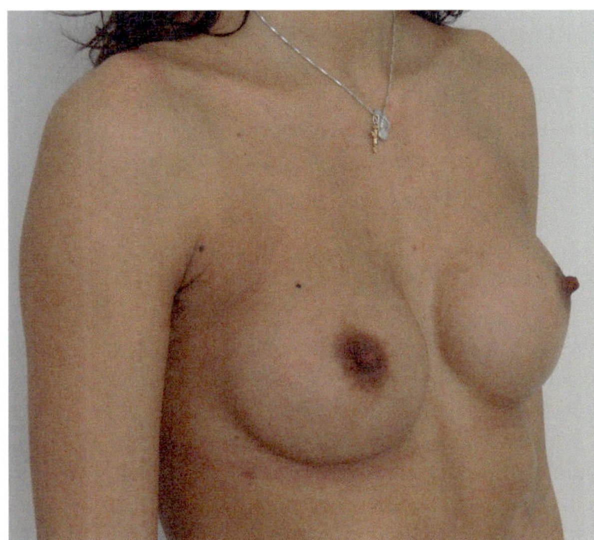

Fig. 9 Postoperative 12 months three quarter right view

augmentation, the pectoralis major is often inadvertently elevated due to the proximity of the origins and unclear muscle plane of separation [15].

Likewise, anomalous pectoralis major slips such as the chondroepitrochlearis can cause medial force vectors when they are overlying the lateral edge of the implant. Literature conclude that overzealous dissection of the medial internal mammary artery perforators and their associated perivascular fibers in the face of an unsuspected thin sternal pectoralis major origin results in sternal muscular dehiscence and reduced medial implant pocket restraint [16].

Thus, it is postulate that the acquired synmastia is due to subpectoral breast augmentation rather than subglandular pocket dissection and that the above events either individually or together contribute to synmastia in virtually all cases. In fact, once begun by dehiscence, the process of Synmastia continues because of the force vectors of the lateralized pectoralis major muscle [15].

Finally, we present our approach based on understanding of the anatomic basis of synmastia putting in evidence our correction that is based on implant pocket exchange from subpectoral positioning to prepectoral one. The subglandular new pocket allows a safe positioning avoiding eventual failure of the repair; we reinforce the new medial limit of the pocket by using single subdermal to periosteum single stiches as described; moreover the new pocket is performed respecting the smaller implant size.

Literature presents a lot of techniques for synmastia repair such as reattaching muscle and pectoralis fascia to the sternum periosteum with or without the use of acellular dermal matrices (ADM) as added support; ADM, as described, is used to repair the medial capsulorrhaphy line protecting the pocket from the maximum weight of the implants [9]. Others suggest using the previous capsule as additional support and creating a neosubpectoral pocket by capsule flaps feeling that the implant should remain under the muscle; in such situations, the capsular flaps are used to prevent migration of the implant after defining of the midline with capsulorrhaphy [3–7, 9, 17, 18].

We report our experience performing synmastia repair as described; we underline the safeness of the technique due to pleasant and long last results; moreover until now, we have seen no recurrences or major complications after our currently recommended and postoperative care.

6 Conclusion

We present our approach for synmastia repair after breast augmentation. The method is simple, reliable, fast, and easy to reproduce allowing pleasant long last results without perioperative major complications or recalcitrant cases.

As elsewhere in surgery, for the management of postaugmentation synmastia, an ounce of prevention is worth a pound of cure. Stated in literature that iatrogenic synmastia is quite always reported after submuscular breast augmentation, we advocate primary breast augmentation by using subglandular implant positioning with a proper implant selection and an accurate pocket dissection.

Our previous studies in the field of breast surgery [19] put in evidence the reliability and efficacy of the prepectoral implant positioning leaving the submuscular pocket only in selected really skinny and undernourished patients.

References

1. Spence RJ, Feldman JJ, Ryan JJ. Synmastia: the problem of medial confluence of the breasts. Plast Reconstr Surg. 1984;73:261.
2. Fredricks S. Medial confluence of the breast. Plast Reconstr Surg. 1985;75:283.
3. Kanhai RC, Hage JJ, Karim RB, et al. Exceptional presenting conditions and outcome of augmentation mammoplasty in male-to-female transsexuals. Ann Plast Surg. 1999;43:476.
4. Bostwick J. Plastic and reconstructive surgery of the breast. 2nd ed. St. Louis: Quality Medical Publishing; 2000.
5. Codner MA, Cohen AT, Hester TR. Complications in breast augmentation: prevention and correction. Clin Plast Surg. 2001;28:587.
6. Chasan PE. Breast capsulorrhaphy revisited: a simple technique for complex problems. Plast Reconstr Surg. 2005;115:296; discussion 302.
7. Becker H, Shaw KE, Kara M. Correction of synmastia using an adjustable implant. Plast Reconstr Surg. 2005;115:2124.
8. Spear SL, Little JW. Breast capsulorrhaphy. Plast Reconstr Surg. 1988;81:274.
9. Baxter RA. Intracapsular allogenic dermal grafts for breast implant-related problems. Plast Reconstr Surg. 2003;112:1692; discussion 1697.
10. de Vita R, Buccheri EM, Villanucci A, et al. Breast asymmetry, classification, and algorithm of treatment: our experience. Aesthet Plast Surg. 2019;43:1439.
11. Auclair E, Anavekar N. Combined use of implant and fat grafting for breast augmentation. Clin Plast Surg. 2015;42(3):307.
12. Spear SL, Majidian A. Immediate breast reconstruction in two stages using textured, integrated-valve tissue ex- panders and breast implants: a retrospective review of 171 consecutive breast reconstructions from 1989 to 1996. Plast Reconstr Surg. 1998;101:53.
13. Sanchez ER, Howland N, Kaltwasser K, et al. Anatomy of the sternal origin of the pectoralis major: implications for subpectoral augmentation. Aesthet Surg J. 2014;34(8):1179.
14. Sanchez ER, Sanchez R, Moliver C. Anatomic relationship of the pectoralis major and minor muscles: a cadaveric study. Aesthet Surg J. 2014;34(2):258.
15. Kalaria SS, Henderson J, Moliver CL. Iatrogenic synmastia: causes and suggested repair technique. Aesthet Surg J. 2019;39(8):863.
16. Lipman A, Strauss E. Treatment of pectoralis major muscle ruptures. Bull Hosp Jt Dis. 2016;74:63.
17. Spear SL, Bogue DP, Thomassen JM. Synmastia after breast augmentation. Plast Reconstr Surg. 2006;118(7 Suppl):171S.
18. Yoo G, Lee PK. Capsular flaps for the management of malpositioned implants after augmentation mammoplasty. Aesthet Plast Surg. 2010;34(1):111.
19. de Vita R, Buccheri EM, Villanucci A, et al. Breast reconstruction actualized in nipple-sparing mastectomy and direct-to-implant, prepectoral polyurethane positioning: early experience and preliminary results. Clin Breast Cancer. 2019;19(2):e358.

Silicone Implant Rupture

Alberto O. Rancati, Claudio Angrigiani, Marcelo Irigo,
Julio Dorr, Juan Acquaviva, Agustin Rancati,
and Maurizio Bruno Nava

1 Background

Breast augmentation is a surgical procedure in which a saline or silicone implant is placed retroglandular or retropectoral in the breast. It can be performed for cosmetic augmentation, reconstruction after mastectomy, or to correct congenital malformations. Approximately 3.5 million people in the United States have breast implants. A possible complication after breast augmentation is implant rupture, which can be intracapsular or extracapsular. The body creates a fibrous capsule scar as a normal reaction to the foreign implant. Intracapsular ruptures refer to implant ruptures that occur within this fibrous capsule, whereas extracapsular ruptures involve extravasation of the silicone gel outside of the fibrous capsule into the surrounding tissues. It is notable that there can be no extracapsular rupture without an intracapsular rupture.

There is a distinction between old silicone prosthesis and new, cohesive silicone prosthesis. In most cases, cohesive silicone will not spread to the surrounding tissue.

Rupture is a long-recognized complication of breast implantation. Retrospective studies about explanted ruptured breast implants that have been approved by the United states (US) and Canada revealed that sharp instrument-induced damage and damage during implantation contribute to the largest number of implant ruptures [1, 2].

2 Etiology

Breast implant durability is an important issue for surgeons, patients, and regulators, such as the Food and Drug Administration (FDA).

A. O. Rancati (✉) · C. Angrigiani · M. Irigo · J. Dorr · J. Acquaviva · A. Rancati
Instituto Oncologico Henry Moore, Universidad de Buenos Aires, Buenos Aires, Argentina

M. B. Nava
University of Milan, Milan, Italy

© Springer Nature Switzerland AG 2022
R. de Vita (ed.), *Aesthetic Breast Augmentation Revision Surgery*,
https://doi.org/10.1007/978-3-030-86793-5_7

Many breast implant manufacturers agree that breast implants are not considered lifetime devices because they may rupture or deflate. Ruptures can occur at any time after surgery, but are more likely to transpire several years after implantation.

3 Identified Rupture Factors

As communicated by Leiden Mentor facility to the authors, on a microscopic study performed on retrieved implants, ruptures can happen for various reasons (Figs. 1, 2, 3, 4, 5, and 6)

- Accidental instrument damage during surgery
- Closed capsulotomy
- Puncture damage due to biopsy or collection
- Folds
- Trauma
- Compression during mammogram
- Manufacturing defects
- Altered thickness of the shell of the implant
- Damage during implantation or explantation

4 Detecting Implant Rupture

Many methods have been used to detect implant rupture and estimate its incidence. Most ruptures are silent and detectable only by certain imaging techniques, such as magnetic resonance imaging (MRI), which is the current gold standard. High-resolution ultrasound is another feasible imaging technique that is being evaluated in some new studies [3]. Patient examinations merely account for approximately 30% of the rupture detected by MRI [4]. Consequently, reports of rupture incidence

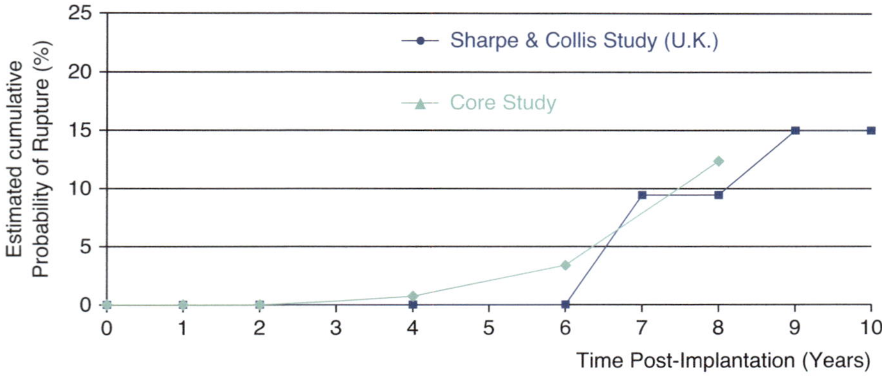

Fig. 1 Damage for instrumental pressure, without peripherical stress

Fig. 2 Shell damage by localized pressure, with signs of peripheral stress

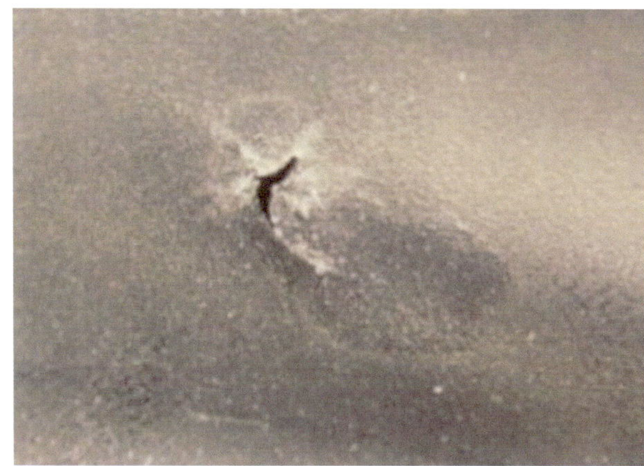

Fig. 3 Patch fault

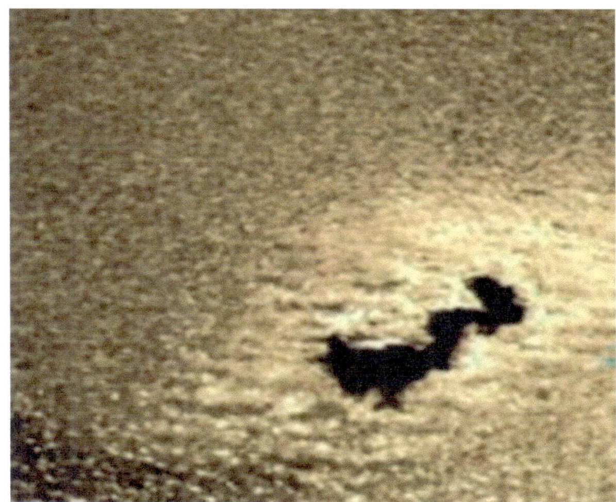

Fig. 4 Damage from cutting scalpel

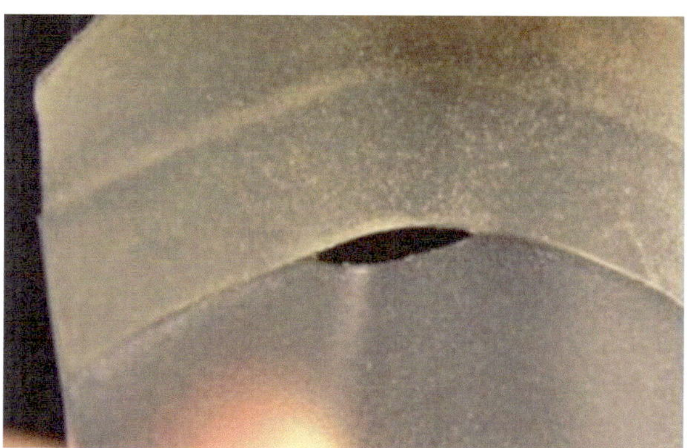

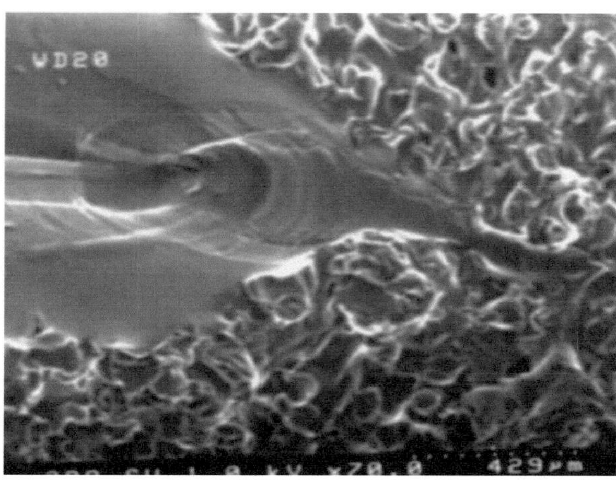

Fig. 5 Tear from needle puncture

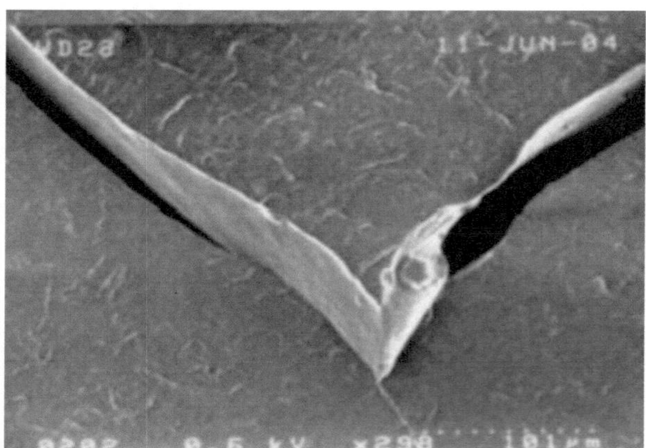

Fig. 6 A typical pattern of damage caused by puncturing

that do not use imaging modalities, such as MRI or ultrasound, will significantly underestimate the actual rupture rate. For this reason, the rupture incidence rate should not be derived from combined populations of MRI-screened and non-MRI-screened patients. Although reports of product complaints have also been used to assess the incidence of rupture, such reports represent only a fraction of the actual complications occurring in patients [5].

5   Rupture Rates Increase Over Time

Incidence rates of rupture increase over time following implantation; that is, rupture rates are very low in the first few years after implantation; therefore the time following implantation is particularly important to consider in any reported estimates of rupture rates. An MRI-based study from Denmark [6] reported estimated

Fig. 7 Estimated cumulative incidence of rupture of MemoryGel® implants (primary augmentation)

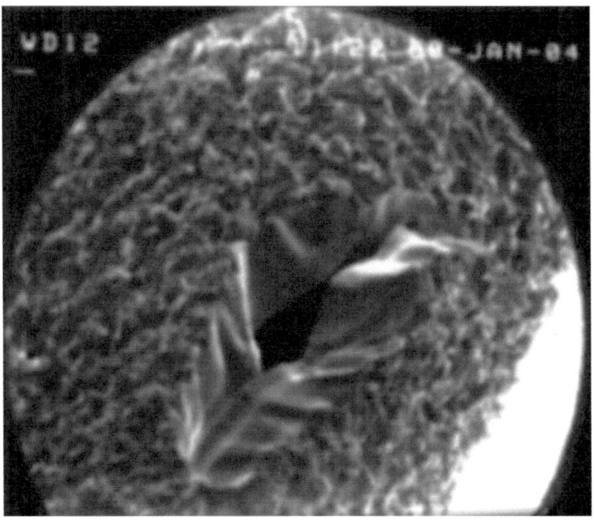

rupture-free rates of 98% 5 years after implantation and 83–85% after 10 years for fifth generation implants that remained intact 3 years after similar results were found in an MRI-based study conducted in the United Kingdom; this study comprised 101 primary augmentation patients with MENTOR® MemoryGel® Breast Implants who presented at the FDA scientific advisory panel hearing in April 2005 [7]. The estimated rupture incidence (by patient) after 10 years was 15.1% (95% confidence interval: 5.6–24.5). Additionally, the current 8-year results from the prospective MemoryGel® Implants Core Study [8] ($n = 202$) align with the findings of the UK study (Fig. 7).

6   Calculating Rupture Rates: All Methods Are Not the Same

When estimating rupture rates from the prospective Core Clinical Study data, follow-up data through the last MRI exam was used, rather than data through the last office visit; this method was used because most ruptures are detected via MRI. However, this method of rupture calculation is not yet standard. Therefore, direct comparisons of rupture rates among studies are not very reliable. Factors such as implant generation, implant type, implant design, and implant shell are important to consider when looking for comparable results.

Available Data Regarding Implant Rupture Rate
- Institute of Medicine of The United States of America (USA)
- Clinical trials conducted at manufacturing facilities
- The Danish Implant Registry
- EU (Allergan study about third generation implants)

- The USA Registry of Breast Implants
- Published literature
- Industry
- The FDA

Implant Rupture Rate (Data from the Danish Implant Registry) [6]
- Implant rupture (%) by implant generation
- First generation 94% to 25 years
- Second generation 52% to 15 years
- Third generation 17% to 10 years–2% to 5 years
- Fourth generation 8% to 11 years [9]
- Fifth generation 1% to 6 years [9]
- Implant rupture depends on time—1 to 4% per year
- The rupture rate was: 5.3 ruptures by every 100 implants/year

The rate of implant rupture depends on the amount of time following implantation, but a rate of 1–4% per year was found in this study. Furthermore, approximately 5.3 ruptures occurred for every 100 implants placed per year.

7 Types of Implant Rupture

There are two types of implant ruptures: silent and symptomatic.

7.1 Silent Rupture of Silicone Gel Breast Implants

A silent rupture occurs when an implant ruptures with no obvious symptoms. This means that neither the patient nor the surgeon would know of the rupture without using diagnostic imaging methods, such as MRI. Because most silicone breast implant ruptures are silent, MRI is recommended 3 years postoperatively, and every 2 years thereafter to screen for rupture. Silent ruptures have increased in frequency due to the use of thicker ("cohesive") silicone gel implants that maintain their shape following rupture; older leaking implants distort after rupturing, making the rupture easier to detect.

7.2 Symptomatic Rupture

A symptomatic rupture occurs when an implant ruptures and produces clinical symptoms that cannot be ignored by the patient, like pain, deformity, or inflammation. To determine the efficiency of a breast implant, it is necessary to determine the primary cause of failure; instrument-related damage seems to be an important factor contributing to implant failure [10]. This evaluation of instrument implant damage can be initiated at different times, including during or before insertion, during implant removal (explantation), or during medical maneuvers (puncture, biopsy, and revision).

Mentor studied and evaluated 240 implants over 10 years and identified the following three causes for implant failure:

1. Iatrogenic user-related problems and surgical damage (22%); these implants had evidence of filtration during surgery and were not implanted (Tables 1, 2, 3, 4, and 5).
2. Rent Unknown Cause (RUC).
3. Not Apparent Etiology Unknown (NAEU) [11].

Implant ruptures can be evaluated by optical microscopy, physical examination, electron microscopy of the rupture site in the explanted implant, and the clinical fatigue test.

Table 1 Modes and causes of implant rupture

RUC and NAEU implant failure modes	N
Localized stress *(presumed cause)*	121
Shell/patch junction	23
Folding flaw	20
Shell/patch delamination	12
Instrument damage	11
Internal patch	3
Combination failures	13
Total	203

RUC Rent Unknown Cause, *NAEU* Not Apparent Etiology Unknown

Table 2 Analysis of retrieved implants

Supplemental analysis of failure modes	# (%) of retrieved devices		
	0–5 years	6–10 years	>10 years
Instrument damage	112 (48%)	5 (13%)	2 (67%)
Localized stress *(presumed cause)*	81 (35%)	16 (40%)	1 (33%)
Shell/patch junction	19 (8%)	4 (10%)	0 (0%)
Folding flaw	10 (4%)	10 (25%)	0 (0%)
Shell/patch delamination	7 (3%)	4 (10%)	0 (0%)
Internal patch	2 (1%)	1 (3%)	0 (0%)
Total	231	40	3

The surface morphology of the retrieved implants was examined using field-emission scanning electron microscopy (SEM) to determine the cause of failure in the first 5 years after implantation, between 6 and 10 years and after 10 years

Table 3 Distribution of failure modes for retrieved devices at 0–5 years ($N = 231$)

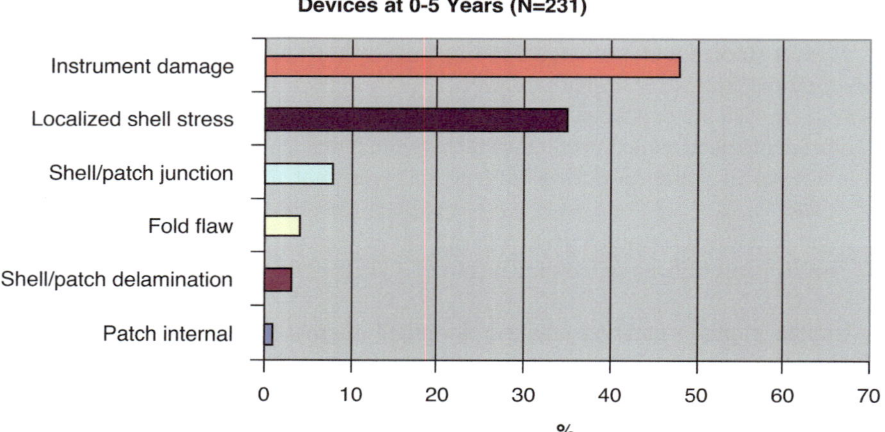

Table 4 Distribution of failure modes for retrieved devices after 6–10 years ($N = 40$)

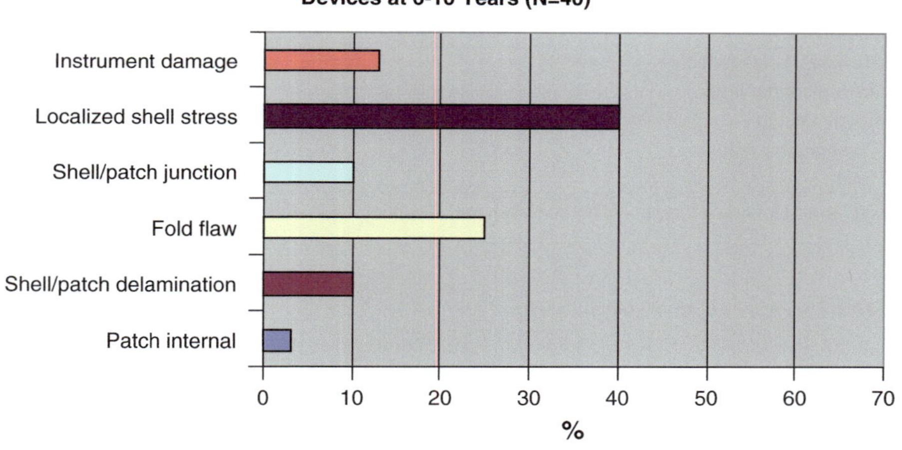

8 Approaches to Minimize Iatrogenic Rupture

These findings have led to a reemphasis on steps to minimize damage, such as:

- Not allowing sharp instruments (i.e., scalpels or needles) to come in contact with the device
- Ensuring that excessive force is not applied to a small area of the shell when inserting the device

Table 5 Distribution of failure mode for retrieved devices after 10 or more years ($N = 3$)

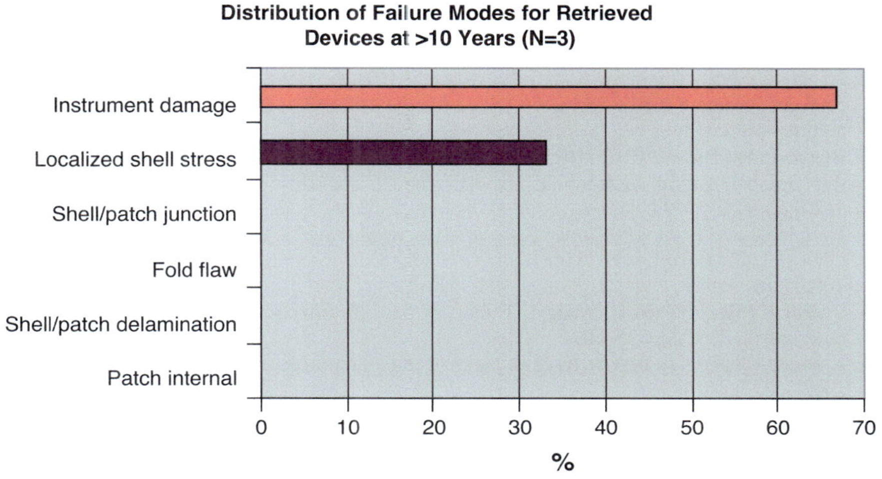

Distribution of Failure Modes for Retrieved Devices at >10 Years (N=3)

Failure mode	%

A horizontal bar chart with the y-axis listing failure modes (Instrument damage, Localized shell stress, Shell/patch junction, Fold flaw, Shell/patch delamination, Patch internal) and the x-axis labeled "%" ranging from 0 to 70. Instrument damage ≈ 67%; Localized shell stress ≈ 33%.

- Making an incision of reasonable length to accommodate the selected style, size, and profile of the implant
- Avoiding creation of wrinkles or folds in the device during implantation

---

9 Conclusions

Implant rupture has long been considered a potential complication of breast implants.

Breast implants are not always lifetime devices and breast implantation is not necessarily a one-time surgery. The most common complications associated with breast implants include reoperation, capsular contracture, asymmetry, and breast pain. Rupture is a less common complication associated with breast implants. The health consequences of a ruptured silicone gel-filled breast implant have not been fully established. MRI screenings are recommended 3 years after initial implant surgery and then every 2 years after to detect silent ruptures. Instrument damage by surgeons seems to be a principal cause of implant rupture in the first 5 years after implantation. The significant contribution of iatrogenic damage to the overall rupture rate suggests that rupture more often may be operator related than device dependent [12].

Disclosures Conflict of interest: Alberto Rancati is worldwide advisor for Mentor implants. Maurizio Bruno Nava is temporary consultant for Allergan. All other authors declare that they have no conflict of interest.

References

1. Health Canada. Summary basis of decision—Mentor MemoryGel® silicone gel-filled breast implants; 2011.
2. Health Canada. Summary basis of decision (SBD) NATRELLETM silicone-filled breast implants—smooth shell with barrier layer and NATRELLETM silicone-filled breast implants-textured shell with barrier layer; 2011.
3. Bengtson BP, Eaves FF 3rd. High-resolution ultrasound in the detection of silicone gel breast implant shell failure: background, in vitro studies, and early clinical results. Aesthet Surg J. 2012;32(2):157–74.
4. Hölmich LR, Fryzek JP, Kjoller K, et al. The diagnosis of silicone breast implant rupture: clinical findings compared with findings at magnetic resonance imaging. Ann Plast Surg. 2005;54(6):583–9.
5. Chernick MR, Poulsen E, Wang Y. Effects of bias adjustment on actuarial survival curves. Drug Info J. 2002;36:595–609.
6. Hölmich LR, Friis S, Fryzek JP, et al. Incidence of silicone breast implant rupture. Arch Surg. 2003;138(7):801–6.
7. Food and Drug Administration (FDA). General and plastic surgery devices panel. 2005. http://www.fda.gov/ohrms/dockets/ac/05/briefing/2005-4101B1-01-08-RUPTURE-MENTOR.pdf. Accessed 21 Feb 2013.
8. Data on file with Mentor Worldwide LLC. MemoryGel® breast implant 9-year core clinical study report; 2011.
9. Heden P, Nava MB, van Tetering JP, et al. Prevalence of rupture in inamed silicone breast implants. Plast Reconstr Surg. 2006;118(2):303–8; discussion 309–312.
10. Brandon HJ, Young VL, Jerina KL, et al. Scanning electron microscopy characterization of surgical instrument damage to breast implants. Plast Reconstr Surg. 2001;108(1):52–61.
11. https://www.fda.gov/ohrms/dockets/ac/05/slides/2005-4101s1_Mentor-P030053.ppt.
12. Handel N, Garcia ME, Wixtrom R. Breast implant rupture: causes, incidence, clinical impact, and management. Plast Reconstr Surg. 2013;132(5):1128–37.

Composite Treatment in Secondary Breast Surgery Infection and Implant Exposure

M. Scheflan, R. Tzur, and R. Wixtrom

1   Introduction

Breast augmentation is one of the most frequently performed procedures in the field of aesthetic plastic surgery. It is the most common cosmetic plastic surgery procedure in United States, with approximately 300,000 performed each year [1].

The risk of surgical site infection (SSI) is present in every surgical procedure and the use of an implant is associated with increased incidence and severity of the infection [2]. Although incidence of post-augmentation mammaplasty infection is generally low, it can be challenging to manage and eradicate. Considerations include onset of symptoms, clinical assessment of stage and severity, antimicrobial treatment in the face of biofilm formation, and timing of surgical intervention.

Periprosthetic infection can manifest itself early, or late following breast augmentation procedures. Infection is often associated with more than just a medical dilemma. Issues such as prolonged hospitalization for intravenous antibiotic treatment, additional surgical interventions, increased costs, patient and surgeon's distress, and potential medicolegal suits prove sometimes to be devastating for patients and often distressing for doctors [3]. The best way to treat infection is to avoid it [4, 5]. Well-established preventive measures and refinements in surgical techniques have been developed in the last two decades [4, 6].

M. Scheflan (✉)
Scheflan Plastic Surgery, Tel Aviv, Israel
e-mail: michael@scheflan.co.il

R. Tzur
Hillel Yaffe Medical Center, Hadera, Israel

R. Wixtrom
Springfield, VA, USA
e-mail: rwixtrom@lscisolutions.com

© Springer Nature Switzerland AG 2022
R. de Vita (ed.), *Aesthetic Breast Augmentation Revision Surgery*,
https://doi.org/10.1007/978-3-030-86793-5_8

Management of post-augmentation infections has evolved over time. Formerly, device removal and delayed replacement were common. More current individual approach includes identification of the offending organism prior to antibiotic initiation, downgrading ("cooling") the stage of infection, early surgical exploration, and implant salvage whenever possible [7–10].

2 Infection Incidence

Incidence of post-augmentation infection is generally quite low, and presents in a bimodal fashion: acute/early in the postoperative period (up to 1 month post-surgery) or with subacute/late onset (more than 1 month post-surgery), with anecdotical cases presenting infections years after augmentation mammaplasty [11].

The most extensive data on the incidence of infection after augmentation mammaplasty is provided by the large, long-term, prospective, multicenter studies conducted by manufacturers to support initial or ongoing regulatory approval [12–17]. The US-based studies (Allergan, Mentor, Sientra) were FDA audited. Table 1 provides a listing of the available cumulative incidence rates (by Kaplan-Meier analysis) of infection in primary augmentation patients from such studies (Note: as these studies were not head-to-head trials, and involved different sets of patients and surgeons, direct rate comparisons between implants are not warranted. The results document both the low incidence of infection in primary augmentation, as well as that the majority of such infections occur within the first year.

In a large-scale international survey conducted in 1970, among 10,941 patients who underwent augmentation mammoplasty by 295 surgeons, the incidence of early and late-onset of post-surgical infections was 1.7% and 0.8%, respectively, with an overall incidence of 2.5% [18]. More contemporary investigations indicate lower incidence: most series showing an incidence of about 1% or less [11, 19–22] with an equal distribution of early- and late-onset infections compared to the older studies; about two thirds of infection occur on the early period, and about one third occur on the late period [11, 23].

Table 1 Cumulative incidence rates of infection in primary augmentation patients

Manufacturer/Implant	Cumulative incidence rate of infection		Number of patients	Ref.
	Through 1 year	Through 10 years		
Allergan round gel	<1%	<1%	455	[12]
Allergan shaped gel	1.5%	1.7%	492	[13, 14]
Mentor round gel	0.7%	0.7%	552	[15]
Mentor shaped gel	0.5%	0.7%	572	[16]
Sientra round and shaped gel	0.5%	0.9%	1116	[17]

3   Risk Factors for Infection

Risk factors for breast implant infection in primary augmentation patients—including patient demographics and comorbidities, intraoperative and postoperative considerations—have been evaluated in a limited number of studies. A UK retrospective analysis of 3000 primary aesthetic breast augmentations of two different surgeons evaluated a number of potential risk factors for infection and other postoperative complications [21]. The risk factors included patient age, incision, implant placement, brand/type of texture, "blind" finger vs. direct view diathermy pocket dissection, use of drains and use of antiseptics/antibiotics for pocket washing. While univariate analysis showed a significant association of infections with the use of drains (increased risk), the use of antibiotics to wash pockets (decreased risk), and imprinted texture prosthesis (decreased risk), multivariate logistic regression analysis did not confirm any of the three variables found to be significant.

A study from the early 1990s included an evaluation of potential risk factors for infection based on 60 reports of early and late mammary implant infections among 54,661 implantations from 73 plastic surgeons [20]. Results specific to augmentation were provided for surface type and showed similar infection rates for smooth, textured, and polyurethane-coated implants (0.06%, 0.16%, and 0.12%, respectively).

The 10-year prospective, multicenter studies mentioned above for Mentor and Allergan also specifically analyzed a number of potential risk factors for infection by Cox regression analyses (the individual factors were similar but not identical between studies). The potential risk factors evaluated included: patient age, race, patient height, patient weight, BMI, smoking status, implant size, time of implantation, general vs. local anesthesia, hospital/surgical facility vs. doctors office, incision site, incision size, implant placement, pocket irrigation (antibiotic/betadine/steroid), surface (texture vs. smooth); and for shaped devices: device height and projection. None of these risk factors for infection were found to be significant by these analyses [14, 16].

Breast incision location (inframammary, periareolar or axillary) does not change the risk for postoperative infection [24].

Other potential predisposing factors for breast implant infection include skin-penetrating injuries, general surgery, dental work, pyoderma, preceding infectious processes, breast trauma, breast massage, breast skin irritation [20], and nipple piercing [25]. Adhesive surgical site dressing could cause a contact dermatitis at the surgical site, and might lead infection of the skin and the implant by Enterobacteriaceae and Pseudomonas aeruginosa [20].

4   Etiology

4.1   Microbiology of the Breast and Possible Sources of Infection

The human breast surface harbors microbial flora, as all other skin surfaces in the human body. The breast also has a diverse endogenous flora, likely derived from the nipple ducts, that includes bacteria found on normal breast skin, as well as bacteria found at other body sites (oral cavity, gastrointestinal tract, respiratory tract, vagina) [26]. Breast ducts allow a passage from the skin surface into deep within the breast tissue [27, 28]. While a notable portion of the breast surface flora is eradicated in the skin preparation process that takes place prior to every surgery, deep breast tissue harbors significant concentrations of endogenous bacteria that is not affected under sterile operating conditions. This endogenous flora could be responsible for contamination of the prosthesis at time of implantation, especially if breast ducts are severed during surgery.

Breast endogenous flora was identified in microbiological cultures studies: tissue cultures were obtained from breast tissue while performing primary operations such as breast augmentation or reduction. Cultures were positive in up to two third of the cases. Coagulase negative staphylococci were shown to be the most common organism isolated (42–53%). Other aerobes included diphtheroids, lactobacillus, D-enterococcus, micrococcus, and alpha-hemolytic streptococcus. Propionibacterium acne (anaerobic diphtheroid) is the most frequent anaerobic bacteria cultured, and in one study grew in 31% of positive cultures. Other anaerobes included peptococcus and Clostridium sporogenes. Fungi species were not isolated from the deep breast tissues [29–31].

Other microbiological studies involved non-infected breasts, during implant exchange surgery, for noninfectious reasons. Cultures were taken from the periprosthetic fluid and/or capsule [32–34] and were positive in 23–50% of cases. In the majority of these studies, most commonly isolated organism was coagulase-negative staphylococci (up to 50% of positive cultures) [33]. In one study, anaerobic diphtheroid was the most common organism isolated (57.5%) [34].

There seem to be no correlation with respect to the type of bacterium and the depth within the breast where cultures were taken [29], but some regions of the breast showed different mean bacterial concentrations: peri areolar region demonstrates bacterial concentration five times higher than that at the inframammary fold region. The latter site demonstrated bacterial counts that were four times higher than those in the axillary region (tail of the breast) [30].

Other possible sources of infection may be related to surgical technique and operation environment. Improper presurgical skin preparation and/or sterile cover as well as any breach in the sterile technique during the operation might contaminate the surgical field and expose the implant pocket to the patients or surgical staff skin flora. A prospective randomized controlled trial of disposable versus reusable gowns and drapes in implant-based breast reconstruction points to reduced infection with the use of disposable gowns [35].

Possible source of infection are hairs and dandruffs from the surgical staff head and facial hair including eyebrows. Failure to exchange surgical tools and gloves and employ the no-touch technique when handling the Implant might expose the patient to unnecessary risk of infection. The surgeon should minimize the use of multiple implants and/or suction drains in primary breast augmentation, and possibly sizers, as there is some evidence these may represent potential sources of infection.

The operation room air contains bacteria-carrying particles that might contaminate the surgical field. A faulty ventilation system or filters will increase particles concentration per cubic meter and thus the potential for deep surgical site infection (SSI) [36].

Also, high flow of human traffic in and out of the OR has been shown to increase the number of bacterial colony-forming units in the room air significantly, and thus should be limited [37].

In late infections, sources may be diverse. Late infections occurring months or years following breast augmentation are commonly caused by secondary bacteremia sourcing from infection in another organ (e.g., peritonitis, cystitis, hidradenitis, UTI, URTI) or an invasive procedure at a location other than the breasts (e.g., oral cavity and dental procedures) [38].

4.2   Common Bacterial Pathogens in Clinically Infected Implants

As previously outlined, presence of various type of bacteria can be found around up to 50% of breast implants, as was shown by studies exploring periprosthetic bacterial flora in non-clinically infected breasts. Nevertheless, only a minority of implanted breasts develop a clinically apparent infection. Thus, overt infection is a multifactorial process. Aside from the presence of bacteria, other factors play a role in periprosthetic infection: bacterial type and load, type of surgery and surgical technique (e.g., cosmetic vs. reconstructive), local tissue factors (e.g., perfusion), host factors and comorbidities and patient susceptibility.

The pathogenesis of infections around breast implants involves an initial phase of bacterial adherence to other cells and the implant surface using cell wall proteins, and secretion of an extracellular polymeric substance, which forms somewhat of a barrier between the bacterial microcolonies and extracellular environment [39]. Ultimately, a mature biofilm is formed. Bacteria embedded in those 3-dimensional biofilm structures are often hard to detect and resistant to antimicrobial agents despite in vitro susceptibility. The lack of a microcirculation in the implanted material and impaired neutrophil function further enhance the host to develop a fully blown infection [23]. Over time the biofilm might reach critical mass over the contaminated implant, which induces a host inflammatory reaction, and can lead to ultimate failure—requiring explantation [4].

Although the odds for infection are inherently higher in the reconstructive population vs. cosmetic population, the microbiology of placing an implant into a pocket adjacent to breast tissues is similar, with skin flora being a common culprit [40].

The most common bacterial pathogens in clinically infected implants, as identified by several microbiological studies, are in descending frequency: Gram-positive bacteria, particularly Staphylococcus aureus and Staphylococcus epidermidis, followed by Gram-negative bacteria (Pseudomonas aeruginosa most common in group, Escherichia coli, Proteus mirabilis, Streptococci A and B, enterobacteria), Streptococci A and B, and anaerobic bacteria [20, 21, 41–43]. Some researchers reported polymicrobial infection [43].

Methicillin-resistant S. aureus infection (MRSA) was described as a possible and uprising pathogen, mainly in postimplant-based breast reconstruction infection [41, 44]. It was associated with poor salvage outcome [44].Late Klebsiella pneumoniae infection has also been reported [45].

Other less common pathogens are: nontuberculous mycobacteria, are responsible for delayed onset and indolent infections [10, 46, 47] and demand special investigations such as acid-fast stains and mycobacterial culture ordered. One should note that the sign and symptoms in these patients may vary significantly in onset and presentation and that they are hard to detect and difficult to treat.

## 5	Preventive Measures

Excellent surgical technique is a critical element of reducing the incidence of infections in breast augmentation. Most device-associated infections are likely to originate from contamination at the time of implantation.

It is also important to recognize that while implant contamination at the time of implantation may lead to the device-associated infections that are the focus of this chapter, it may also result in subclinical periprosthetic bacterial infection that is a well-established etiologic factor in potentiating the development of capsular contracture [28]. Also, data suggest that chronic bacterial biofilm inflammation may in part be responsible for the development of breast implant-associated anaplastic large-cell lymphoma (ALCL), possibly through incitement of substantial T-cell activation and response [4, 6, 48], although limited conflicting findings have also been published [49].

The occurrence of periprosthetic breast infections may be minimized by adhering to strict surgical techniques, such as the 14-point plan described by Deva, Adams, and Vickery (2013, Box 1) [4], which was further extended recently by Jewell et al. [50].

> **Box 1 14-Point Plan to Minimize Periprosthetic Bacterial Load) [4]**
> 1. Use intravenous antibiotic prophylaxis at the time of anesthetic induction
> 2. Avoid periareolar incisions; these have been shown in both laboratory and clinical studies to lead to a higher rate of capsule contracture as the pocket dissection is contaminated directly by bacteria within the breast tissue
> 3. Use nipple shields to prevent spillage of bacteria into the pocket
> 4. Avoid blunt finger dissection and perform careful atraumatic dissection to minimize devascularized tissue
> 5. Perform careful hemostasis
> 6. Avoid dissection into the breast parenchyma. The use of a dual-plane, subfascial pocket has anatomic advantages
> 7. Perform pocket irrigation with triple antibiotic solution or betadine

8. Use an introduction sleeve whenever possible and available
9. Use new instruments and drapes, and change surgical gloves prior to handling the implant
10. Immerse the implant in antibiotic solution prior to opening and minimize the time of implant opening and exposure to operating room air
11. Minimize repositioning and replacement of the implant
12. Use a layered closure
13. Avoid using a drainage tube, which can be a potential site of entry for bacteria
14. Use antibiotic prophylaxis to cover subsequent procedures that breach skin or mucosa

Jewell et al. offered additional Steps to Diminish Risk of Microbial Contamination beyond Deva's 14 Steps [50], among which:

MRSA screening by nasal swab at preoperative visit; if positive decontamination with PI or mupirocin

Avoidance of staff/anesthesia personnel turnovers (no in and out operating room traffic)

When using a sizer implant, coat it with Betadine before insertion into pocket with an insertion sleeve

If drains are used, have a "no-touch" drain insertion technique; chlorhexidine (CHG)-impregnated drain dressing patches

Antimicrobial-coated sutures utilize an insertion sleeve when available

Surgeon/operating room staff avoidance of swimming pools or Jacuzzi pools before surgery (atypical mycobacteria out-break) (41)

Surgeon avoidance of healthcare environments where surgeon could be contaminated with Gram+ or Gram− organisms before surgery, e.g., wound clinic, infected surgical case, burn unit, etc. Adherence to standardized to breast augmentation practices that include infection prevention measures has been shown to result in significantly lower postoperative complications [6, 51].

Barr et al. performed an extensive literature review encompassing a wide variety of possible surgical site infection prevention methods. They presented summaries of the available aseptic methods and their validity to use as guidelines for infection prevention strategies in implant-based breast reconstruction. The infection prevention methods were categorized and evaluated, and a recommendation made with regard to its use. Methods were defined as "suggested" if the evidence supporting it were weak or insufficient (Box 2), and "recommended" if the evidence supporting it were sufficient (Box 3). Methods were categorized as "not recommended" if there was very weak evidence or no evidence supporting it (Box 4) [5].

> **Box 2 Barr et al. Suggested Infection Preventive Methods [5]**
> Solution type for skin preparation: alcoholic chlorhexidine
> Laminar air flow and ultraclean ventilation
> Avoid use of drains

> **Box 3 Barr et al. Recommended Infection Preventive Methods [5]**
> - Preoperative methicillin-sensitive and -resistant S. aureus screening and treatment
> - Use of prophylactic antibiotics
>
>   Patient warming
>
> - Minimization of theatre staffing levels
> - Double glove use
> - Operative duration
> - Implant and pocket washing

> **Box 4 Infection Preventive Methods with No Specific Recommendation According to Barr et al. [5]**
> Antibacterial showering preoperatively
> Use of nipple shields
> Implant type
> Grade of operating surgeon
> Incision site

With respect to the use of nipple shields, the Barr analysis did not appear to consider the more recent findings of a controlled Finnish study by Giordano et al. [52] that identified a statistically significant reduction in capsular contracture, presumably due to reduced introduction of bacteria into the surgical pocket.

6 The Role of Static Charges Around Implants

Breast implants shells are made of silicone polymer that possess electrostatic charges on its outer surface area. Those charges create an electrostatic field that attracts oppositely charged particles onto the outer surface area of the implant. When a fresh out-of-the-package implant is brought near a lightweight particle such as thin paper strips, one can observe attraction of the particles to the implant as a result of the electrostatic field [53]. Thus, during an implant breast surgery, the implant is theoretically exposed to another possible way of contamination: free floating particles in the operating room air, which might be attracted to the implant before inserted to the pocket. If those particles contain bacteria, this might lead to an infection and/or capsular contracture. The use of laminar airflow in operating theatres may reduce but not eliminate the particulate count and thermal plume within the operating theatre and inadvertent deposition of airborne microscopic particulate matter on medical devices is possible [54].

In a yet to be published study done by our group, breast implants electrostatic charges were measured by a static sensor. We recorded charges of up to 20.000 V around the plastic package that houses the breast implant. When the implant was removed from its package, the electrostatic field dropped by 50% or less, and when implant was wetted with saline, the electrostatic charges measured dropped to almost zero. We then hovered a sterile, smooth or textured implant, dry or wet, fresh out of the package, 2 cm over colonies of skin bacteria, and then took serial microbiologic cultures. Preliminary results showed no or scant bacterial growth on dry implant surfaces, abundant growth on saline wet surfaces, and no growth on triple antibiotic wetted implant surfaces.

The question whether or not bacteria attracted to strong electrostatic field around breast implants remained unanswered in our pilot study. Nevertheless, we [MS, RT] routinely inject the triple antibiotic solution, containing betadine diluted 1:1, directly through the sealed paper cover of the sterile package, before opening it, then shake it gently. This quick and easy maneuver will neutralize the static charges around the implant and temporarily coat the implant with a film of antibiotic solution during insertion into the breast pocket.

7   Antibiotic Protocols to Reduce Infection

In the era of increasing awareness of antibiotic-resistant organisms, the use of prophylactic antibiotics in cosmetic breast implant surgery remains controversial. The two key elements of breast implant placement are the use of a foreign body (implant) and the presence of bacterial flora in the breast. In light of the data, showing that deep breast tissue harbors significant concentrations of bacteria in breast ducts [28–30], one might argue that breast surgery is better categorized as "clean contaminated" surgery, rather than "clean." The National Institute for Health and Clinical Excellence (NICE) recommends the use of systemic prophylactic antibiotics in clean surgery involving a prosthesis [55].

It seems that prospective studies comparing patients undergoing breast augmentation surgery with or without prophylactic antibiotic treatment have insufficient group sizes to unequivocally determine the need for prophylactic antibiotics. Those studies have small sample sizes for intervention and control group, compared to the low incidences of postoperative infections reported in literature, and did not show any difference in rates of infection between the two groups [11, 56].

In a large retrospective study done by Khan et al., three groups of patients undergoing breast augmentation surgery compared according to their prophylaxis protocol: single intravenous first generation cephalosporin dose, single intravenous dose plus an oral dose for 24 h, or a single intravenous dose plus an oral course for 5 days. The incidence of infection was lowest with a single perioperative dose of intravenous antibiotic compared with a combination of intravenous and oral antibiotics. They concluded that a single dose of intravenous antibiotic is adequate for prophylaxis in breast augmentation surgery, and the extra duration of antibiotic cover does not result in reduced superficial or periprosthetic infections [7].

A large retrospective survey of 1487 plastic surgeons and about 40,000 breast augmentations found 254 infections (0.64%). In the prophylaxis group infection rate was 0.42%, significantly lower compared with 0.87% in the control group with no prophylaxis antibiotic treatment [57].

As for the duration of prophylactic antibiotic treatment, a large retrospective study evaluated postoperative 3 day antibiotic treatment after primary and secondary breast augmentation. The data suggest that there was no reduction in the overall rate of total complications, infection, or capsular contracture with postoperative prophylactic antibiotic treatment for either primary or secondary cosmetic breast augmentation [58].

We [MS, RT] give a single dose of intravenous first- or second-generation cephalosporin before starting anesthetic procedures. Long surgical time may require an additional intraoperative dose of antibiotic, in accordance with the specific antibiotic half-life duration. In patients with allergies to beta-lactam antibiotics, a non-beta-lactam antibiotic with adequate spectrum is recommended.

8 Signs and Symptoms

Acute periprosthetic infections are usually associated with breast erythema, evolving pain, tenderness, and fever [34, 42]. Onset of acute infections occur between first postoperative day and sixth postoperative week [18, 20, 23]. The average onset time is 10–12 days after surgery [3, 18].

Toxic shock syndrome has been reported to occur following breast implant surgery and most commonly associated with Staphylococcus aureus bacteria. It is a rapidly evolving, life-threatening condition, requiring immediate surgical exploration and removal of the implant followed with antibiotic treatment [59–61]. It can present clinically as sore throat accompanied by high fever, diarrhea, lethargy, myalgia, and a rash later accompanied or followed with hypotension and acute respiratory distress syndrome as described by Barnett [62]. The symptoms may begin earlier than a usual surgical site acute infection: first signs of toxic shock syndrome may appear in the first 12–24 h after surgery. Surgical site and operative wound appearance are rarely impressive, and neither inflammation nor purulence may be present. Although no local signs of infection are present, the patient might suffer from a fulminant, life-threatening sepsis [27, 63].

Periprosthetic late infection occurs after more than 6 weeks of surgery. Onset time of late infection extends from a few months to several years after surgery. This onset time late infection is different for saline implants and silicone implants: saline implant infections occur within 8 weeks (on average 4 weeks), while silicone implant infections occur within 26 weeks (on average 13 weeks) [3]. The earlier onset of saline implant infections may be linked to contamination during implant filling [41].

Late infection usually results from a bacteremia. This bacteremia may be secondary to an injury or an invasive procedure, at a location other than the breast [18, 20, 45, 64, 65]. Similar to other temporary or permanent artificial implants placed within body tissues, breast implants may act as a surface attractive to bacterial colonization, particularly when bloodstream infection occurs. Therefore, as early as possible systemic antibiotics is promptly and aggressively initiated in order to limit these rare secondary infections. Likewise, invasive dental surgical procedures, especially when performed under septic conditions, should be accompanied with antibiotic prophylaxis if possible [3, 27]. Late infections may present only with vague breast pain with or without inflammatory skin changes [66], or with focal symptoms, such as a nonhealing surgical site, redness, drainage, dehiscence, or extrusion of the implant [23]. Nontuberculous mycobacterial infections are important to consider in patients with acute or subacute symptoms with breast swelling or fullness sensation, signs of inflammation that can be mild or even absent, with or without fever, serous or sero-purulent drainage that is culture-negative on routine bacterial cultures, and no response to first line antibiotic treatment [10, 23, 46, 47]. Recommended treatment for mycobacterial implant infection is explantation and long-term supplemented antibiotic treatment [10].

9   Diagnosis and Treatment

Diagnosis of breast implant infection is largely clinical. The diagnosis relies mainly on local and/or systemic manifestations. As noted, signs and symptoms might include complains of discomfort and tension, change in breast shape, pain, local redness and swelling, tenderness, fever, drainage, dehiscence, and implant exposure. The surgeon must address urgently signs of severe systemic infection such as high fever, hypotension, or other signs of sepsis. In those cases, treatment should be aggressive and without any delay.

As noted previously, toxic shock syndrome is also possible following breast implant surgery (as well as other surgery not including implants). It typically presents soon after implant placement, with signs of sepsis such as fever, hypotension, rash, nausea, vomiting, diarrhea, and eventually multiorgan system failure. In those cases, signs of infection at the operative site are usually absent, and a high index of suspicion is needed for proper diagnosis and treatment. Patients presenting with signs of sepsis soon after implant placement should be treated with prompt removal of the prosthesis [23].

Infection must be distinguished between red breast syndrome: a non-infectious, self-limited erythema of breast after the use of acellular dermal matrix (ADM) [67]. A recent study provided significant evidence that red breast syndrome is likely attributable to endotoxin present within the ADM at the time of implantation [68].

Blood work should be obtained routinely and include complete blood count, biochemistry panel and concentration of c-reactive protein (CRP) or erythrocyte sedimentation rate (ESR). Leukocytosis, neutrophilia, high ESR, and high blood concentration of CRP raise the suspicion of more serious, systemic infection, but are usually not reliable indicators in the immediate postoperative period.

Identification of the pathogen is imperative when possible. It will facilitate accurate antibiotic treatment and prevent the appearance of resistant bacteria strains. Where available, newer molecular methods of microbial analysis that are based on detection of nucleic acid sequences, rather than requiring culturing, are more sensitive and can detect a much broader range of potential pathogens [69]. Cultures, or specimens for molecular microbiology analysis, must be obtained when indicated, from wound, any drainage and blood, before the initiation of any antibiotic treatment.

The use of ultrasonography in the suspected implant breast infection is not unanimously agreed upon. Ultrasonography imaging quality is highly dependent on the operator and its results cannot be uniformly addressed. The absence of a fluid collection on ultrasound does not rule out implant infection. In some cases, peri prosthetic fluid might not show in ultrasonography imaging, although actually exists as proven at the time of operation. When periprosthetic fluid is recognized by ultrasonography, it is usually impossible to determine if the fluid is infected. Nevertheless, when there is no indication for surgical exploration, it is recommended to aspirate periprosthetic fluid with the guidance of ultrasonography for culture purposes [3, 27, 66]. Care should be taken not to damage the implant.

There are no randomized, controlled trials of infection of breast implant that compared conservative treatment (e.g., antibiotic treatment) with surgical intervention (e.g., implant exchange or removal). Historically, management of breast implant infection has included systemic antimicrobial therapy and implant removal in most cases [66]. Today, breast implant infection approach has changed, and breast implants can be salvaged in selective cases.

Treatment rationales are:

Sings of severe sepsis or toxic shock syndrome will prompt surgical exploration.

Redness, pain, tenderness, and swelling, with no signs of fever, discharge, or extrusion, will be considered as level 1 infection (Fig. 1) and will be treated with oral antibiotics. If there is no adequate response after 48 hours of treatment, treatment will be continued parentally.

Redness, pain, tenderness, swelling, and fever will be considered as level 2 infection (Fig. 2) and will be treated with parenteral antibiotics. For cases of complete response, treatment can be continued orally with close follow-up. For no response or partial response—surgical exploration is in order.

Redness, pain, tenderness, swelling, fever and discharge or implant exposure will be considered as level 3 infection and will be treated with surgical exploration.

Exposure of breast implant will be treated with surgical exploration.

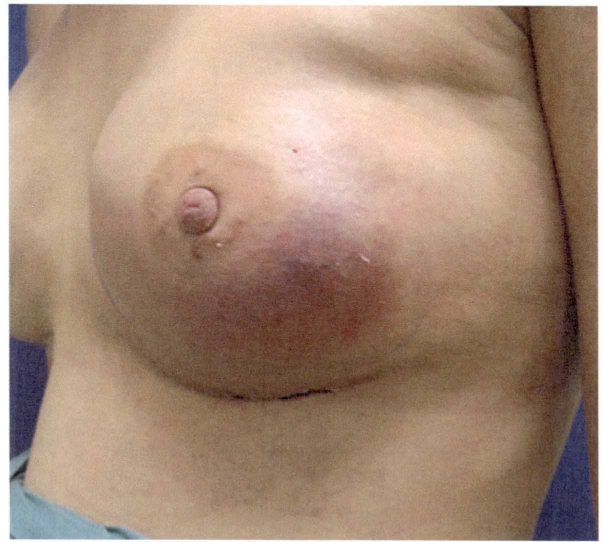

Fig. 1 A 34-year-old patient, 6 months after implant surgery of left breast, presented with pain, redness, swelling, and tenderness: Level 1 periprosthetic infection

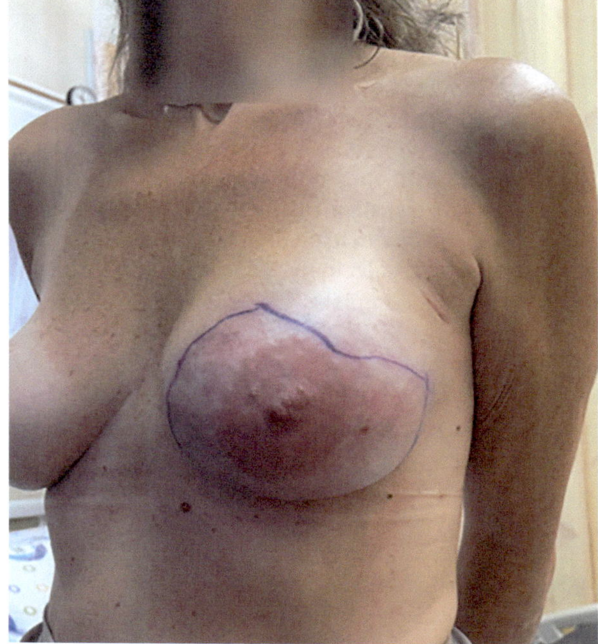

Fig. 2 A 51-year-old patient, 2 years after silicone implant surgery of left breast, presented with systemic fever, pain, redness, swelling, and tenderness: Level 2 periprosthetic infection

A lack of improvement following a prolonged empiric therapy and implant removal should raise suspicion of late or rare infections.

Treatment summary and algorithm is presented in Fig. 3.

Surgical exploration: For stable patients, surgical exploration will be indicated for Level 1 and level 2 infections, which did not respond to parenteral antibiotic

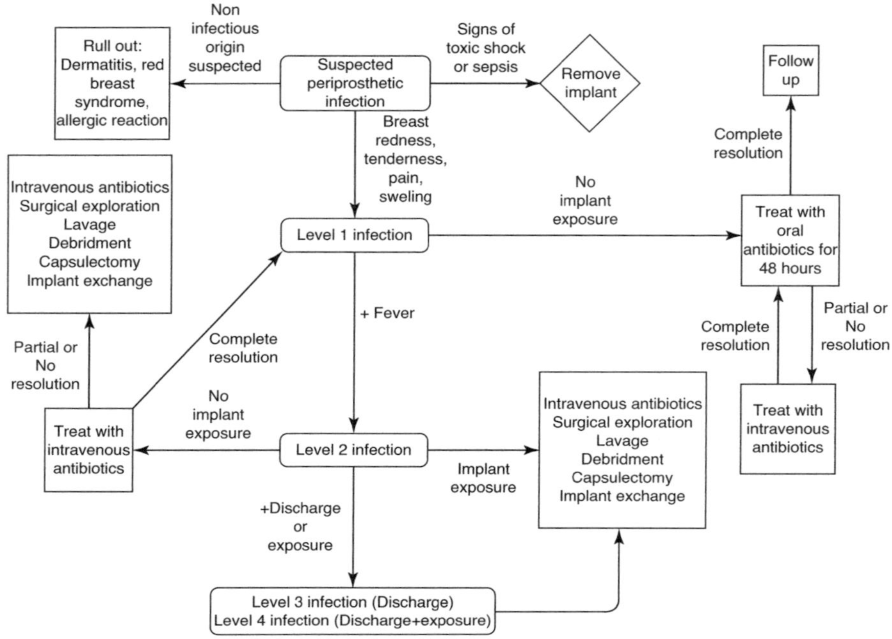

Fig. 3 Periprosthetic infection treatment algorithm

treatment, for level 3 infection and for implant extrusion. The possibility of implant salvage will be clinically evaluated during the exploration: for implant pockets that contain puss or substantial amount of granulation tissue, salvage is not recommended and implant explantation is in order after proper lavage, debridement, and in some cases capsulectomy. Closure will be done over close suction drain and replacement of the implant will be postponed for 6 months. In the absence of puss or granulation tissue, implant will be replaced after proper lavage, debridement and in some cases also capsulectomy and coverage with local flaps, and closure over close suction drain. It is important to culture any fluid present in the implant pocket and obtain a tissue sample for bacterial culture during exploration.

Wound dehiscence with implant exposure is not always accompanied by clinical infection and may be a result of an increase of intracapsular pressure or low skin perfusion. In those cases, the implant is nevertheless considered as contaminated, and surgical exploration with implant exchange is a safe treatment modality.

For patients with level 2 or level 3 infection, with good response to parenteral antibiotic treatment, the next step of treatment is debatable. Oral antibiotic and close follow-up is an acceptable option for complete responders with no residual signs of any clinical infection, especially in the level 2 group. The major drawback of this treatment method is the expected biofilm left on the implant, and supposedly higher chance of infection recurrence and capsular contracture. A safer approach will be surgical exploration, cultures, lavage, debridement implant exchange and closure over close suction drains. In the few investigations done on this topic, it seems that in the presence of periprosthetic severe infection, or periprosthetic implant infection and extrusion, 50–70% rates of implants were explanted [8, 9, 44, 70].

Whenever in doubt, we advocate surgical exploration as the safest treatment option. However, if complete response with no residual signs of infection was observed, we allow oral antibiotic treatment and close follow-up.

10   In Closing

Breast augmentation using implants is the most common cosmetic surgical procedure in the United States, and like any other surgery harbors the risk of surgical site infection (SSI). While the incidence is quite low (1.5% or lower), the use of an implant is associated with increased incidence and severity of the infection which may be challenging to manage and eradicate.

Etiology of periprosthetic infection is not merely a presence of bacteria, but rather a multifactorial process involving surgical technique, tissue, and host factors.

Infection must best be prevented by adhering to strict surgical techniques and perioperative guidelines specific to the use of implants. When diagnosing periprosthetic infection, identification of the pathogen before instituting antibiotic treatment is imperative.

Antibiotic treatment may prove insufficient in itself and should be combined with surgical exploration and implant exchange in most all advanced cases.

References

1. (ASPS) ASoPS. Cosmetic plastic surgery statistics 2018. https://www.plasticsurgery.org/documents/News/Statistics/2018/plastic-surgery-statistics-report-2018.pdf.
2. Sugarman B. Infections and prosthetic devices. Am J Med. 1986;81(1a):78–84.
3. Rubino C, Brongo S, Pagliara D, Cuomo R, Abbinante G, Campitiello N, et al. Infections in breast implants: a review with a focus on developing countries. J Infect Dev Ctries. 2014;8(9):1089–95.
4. Deva AK, Adams WP Jr, Vickery K. The role of bacterial biofilms in device-associated infection. Plast Reconstr Surg. 2013;132(5):1319–28.
5. Barr SP, Topps AR, Barnes NL, Henderson J, Hignett S, Teasdale RL, et al. Infection prevention in breast implant surgery—a review of the surgical evidence, guidelines and a checklist. Eur J Surg Oncol. 2016;42(5):591–603.
6. Adams WP Jr, Culbertson EJ, Deva AK, Magnusson MR, Layt C, Jewell ML, et al. Macrotextured breast implants with defined steps to minimize bacterial contamination around the device: experience in 42,000 implants. Plast Reconstr Surg. 2017;140(3):427–31.
7. Khan UD. Breast augmentation, antibiotic prophylaxis, and infection: comparative analysis of 1,628 primary augmentation mammoplasties assessing the role and efficacy of antibiotics prophylaxis duration. Aesthet Plast Surg. 2010;34(1):42–7.
8. Spear SL, Howard MA, Boehmler JH, Ducic I, Low M, Abbruzzesse MR. The infected or exposed breast implant: management and treatment strategies. Plast Reconstr Surg. 2004;113(6):1634–44.

9. Spear SL, Seruya M. Management of the infected or exposed breast prosthesis: a single surgeon's 15-year experience with 69 patients. Plast Reconstr Surg. 2010;125(4):1074–84.
10. Scheflan M, Wixtrom RN. Over troubled water: an outbreak of infection due to a new species of mycobacterium following implant-based breast surgery. Plast Reconstr Surg. 2016;137(1):97–105.
11. Gravante G, Caruso R, Araco A, Cervelli V. Infections after plastic procedures: incidences, etiologies, risk factors, and antibiotic prophylaxis. Aesthet Plast Surg. 2008;32(2):243–51.
12. Adllergan. Directions for use NATRELLE® silicone-filled breast implants and NATRELLE INSPIRA® breast implants smooth & BIOCELL® texture. https://media.allergan.com/acta-vis/actavis/media/allergan-pdf-documents/labeling/natrelleus/siliconeimplants/natrelle-and-inspira-dfu-l034rev12.pdf.
13. administration fad. Summary of safety and effectiveness data allergan gel-filled mammary prosthesis. https://www.accessdata.fda.gov/cdrh_docs/pdf4/P040046b.pdf.
14. Maxwell GP, Van Natta BW, Bengtson BP, Murphy DK. Ten-year results from the Natrelle 410 anatomical form-stable silicone breast implant core study. Aesthet Surg J. 2015;35(2):145–55.
15. Mentor. Product insert data sheet MENTOR® MEMORYGEL™ and MENTOR® MEMORYGEL™ xtra silicone gel breast implants. http://synthes.vo.llnwd.net/o16/LLNWMB8/IFUs/OUS/Mentor/MemoryGel%20Non-CE%20Marked%20ePIDS_Final.pdf.
16. Hammond DC, Canady JW, Love TR, Wixtrom RN, Caplin DA. Mentor contour profile gel implants: clinical outcomes at 10 years. Plast Reconstr Surg. 2017;140(6):1142–50.
17. Inc S. Summary of safety and effectiveness data of Sientra silicone gel-filled breast implants. https://www.accessdata.fda.gov/cdrh_docs/pdf7/p070004b.pdf.
18. De Cholnoky T. Augmentation mammaplasty. Survey of complications in 10,941 patients by 265 surgeons. Plast Reconstr Surg. 1970;45(6):573–7.
19. Kjøller K, Hölmich LR, Jacobsen PH, Friis S, Fryzek J, McLaughlin JK, et al. Epidemiological investigation of local complications after cosmetic breast implant surgery in Denmark. Ann Plast Surg. 2002;48(3):229–37.
20. Brand KG. Infection of mammary prostheses: a survey and the question of prevention. Ann Plast Surg. 1993;30(4):289–95.
21. Araco A, Gravante G, Araco F, Delogu D, Cervelli V, Walgenbach K. Infections of breast implants in aesthetic breast augmentations: a single-center review of 3,002 patients. Aesthet Plast Surg. 2007;31(4):325–9.
22. Handel N, Cordray T, Gutierrez J, Jensen JA. A long-term study of outcomes, complications, and patient satisfaction with breast implants. Plast Reconstr Surg. 2006;117(3):757–67; discussion 68–72.
23. Lalani T. Breast implant infections: an update. Infect Dis Clin N Am. 2018;32(4):877–84.
24. Stutman RL, Codner M, Mahoney A, Amei A. Comparison of breast augmentation incisions and common complications. Aesthet Plast Surg. 2012;36(5):1096–104.
25. Javaid M, Shibu M. Breast implant infection following nipple piercing. Br J Plast Surg. 1999;52(8):676–7.
26. Urbaniak C, Cummins J, Brackstone M, Macklaim JM, Gloor GB, Baban CK, et al. Microbiota of human breast tissue. Appl Environ Microbiol. 2014;80(10):3007–14.
27. Pittet B, Montandon D, Pittet D. Infection in breast implants. Lancet Infect Dis. 2005;5(2):94–106.
28. Galdiero M, Larocca F, Iovene MR, Martora F, Pieretti G, D'Oriano V, et al. Microbial evaluation in capsular contracture of breast implants. Plast Reconstr Surg. 2018;141(1):23–30.
29. Thornton JW, Argenta LC, McClatchey KD, Marks MW. Studies on the endogenous flora of the human breast. Ann Plast Surg. 1988;20(1):39–42.
30. Bartsich S, Ascherman JA, Whittier S, Yao CA, Rohde C. The breast: a clean-contaminated surgical site. Aesthet Surg J. 2011;31(7):802–6.
31. Wixtrom RN, Stutman RL, Burke RM, Mahoney AK, Codner MA. Risk of breast implant bacterial contamination from endogenous breast flora, prevention with nipple shields, and implications for biofilm formation. Aesthet Surg J. 2012;32(8):956–63.

32. Netscher DT, Weizer G, Wigoda P, Walker LE, Thornby J, Bowen D. Clinical relevance of positive breast periprosthetic cultures without overt infection. Plast Reconstr Surg. 1995;96(5):1125–9.
33. Pajkos A, Deva AK, Vickery K, Cope C, Chang L, Cossart YE. Detection of subclinical infection in significant breast implant capsules. Plast Reconstr Surg. 2003;111(5):1605–11.
34. Ahn CY, Ko CY, Wagar EA, Wong RS, Shaw WW. Microbial evaluation: 139 implants removed from symptomatic patients. Plast Reconstr Surg. 1996;98(7):1225–9.
35. Showalter BM, Crantford JC, Russell GB, Marks MW, DeFranzo AJ, Thompson JT, et al. The effect of reusable versus disposable draping material on infection rates in implant-based breast reconstruction: a prospective randomized trial. Ann Plast Surg. 2014;72(6):S165–9.
36. Lidwell OM, Lowbury EJ, Whyte W, Blowers R, Stanley SJ, Lowe D. Airborne contamination of wounds in joint replacement operations: the relationship to sepsis rates. J Hosp Infect. 1983;4(2):111–31.
37. Andersson AE, Bergh I, Karlsson J, Eriksson BI, Nilsson K. Traffic flow in the operating room: an explorative and descriptive study on air quality during orthopedic trauma implant surgery. Am J Infect Control. 2012;40(8):750–5.
38. Basile AR, Basile F, Basile AV. Late infection following breast augmentation with textured silicone gel-filled implants. Aesthet Surg J. 2005;25(3):249–54.
39. Oliveira WF, Silva PMS, Silva RCS, Silva GMM, Machado G, Coelho L, et al. Staphylococcus aureus and Staphylococcus epidermidis infections on implants. J Hosp Infect. 2018;98(2):111–7.
40. Cohen JB, Carroll C, Tenenbaum MM, Myckatyn TM. Breast implant-associated infections: the role of the National Surgical Quality Improvement Program and the local microbiome. Plast Reconstr Surg. 2015;136(5):921–9.
41. Feldman EM, Kontoyiannis DP, Sharabi SE, Lee E, Kaufman Y, Heller L. Breast implant infections: is cefazolin enough? Plast Reconstr Surg. 2010;126(3):779–85.
42. Armstrong RW, Berkowitz RL, Bolding F. Infection following breast reconstruction. Ann Plast Surg. 1989;23(4):284–8.
43. Seng P, Bayle S, Alliez A, Romain F, Casanova D, Stein A. The microbial epidemiology of breast implant infections in a regional referral centre for plastic and reconstructive surgery in the south of France. Int J Infect Dis. 2015;35:62–6.
44. Reish RG, Damjanovic B, Austen WG Jr, Winograd J, Liao EC, Cetrulo CL, et al. Infection following implant-based reconstruction in 1952 consecutive breast reconstructions: salvage rates and predictors of success. Plast Reconstr Surg. 2013;131(6):1223–30.
45. Bernardi C, Saccomanno F. Late Klebsiella pneumoniae infection following breast augmentation: case report. Aesthet Plast Surg. 1998;22(3):222–4.
46. Macadam SA, Mehling BM, Fanning A, Dufton JA, Kowalewska-Grochowska KT, Lennox P, et al. Nontuberculous mycobacterial breast implant infections. Plast Reconstr Surg. 2007;119(1):337–44.
47. Thomas M, D'Silva JA, Borole AJ, Chilgar RM. Periprosthetic atypical mycobacterial infection in breast implants: a new kid on the block! J Plast Reconstr Aesthet Surg. 2013;66(1):e16–9.
48. Khavanin N, Clemens MW, Pusic AL, Fine NA, Hamill JB, Kim HM, et al. Shaped versus round implants in breast reconstruction: a multi-institutional comparison of surgical and patient-reported outcomes. Plast Reconstr Surg. 2017;139(5):1063–70.
49. Walker JN, Hanson BM, Pinkner CL, Simar SR, Pinkner JS, Parikh R, et al. Insights into the microbiome of breast implants and periprosthetic tissue in breast implant-associated anaplastic large cell lymphoma. Sci Rep. 2019;9(1):10393.
50. Jewell ML, Fickas B, Jewell H, Jewell ML. Implant surface options and biofilm mitigation strategies. Plast Reconstr Surg. 2019;144(1S):13s–20s.
51. Santorelli A, Rossano F, Cagli B, Avvedimento S, Ghanem A, Marlino S. Standardized practice reduces complications in breast augmentation: results with the first 290 consecutive cases versus non-standardized comparators. Aesthet Plast Surg. 2019;43(2):336–47.
52. Giordano S, Salmi A. Nipple shields as additional tool to pocket irrigation in reducing capsular contracture after cosmetic breast augmentation. Plast Reconstr Surg. 2014;134(2S):386.

53. Khoo LS, Stevens HP. Preventing electrostatic contamination of breast implants: an effective and simple intraoperative method. Aesthet Surg J. 2017;37(6):731–3.
54. Chow TT, Yang XY. Ventilation performance in operating theatres against airborne infection: review of research activities and practical guidance. J Hosp Infect. 2004;56(2):85–92.
55. Health NCCfWsaCs. Surgical site infection: prevention and treatment of surgical site infection. National Institute for Health and Clinical Excellence (NICE); 2008. http://www.nice.org.uk/nicemedia/live/11743/42378/42378.pdf.
56. Keramidas E, Lymperopoulos NS, Rodopoulou S. Is antibiotic prophylaxis in breast augmentation necessary? A prospective study. Plast Surg (Oakv). 2016;24(3):195–8.
57. Clegg HW, Bertagnoll P, Hightower AW, Baine WB. Mammaplasty-associated mycobacterial infection: a survey of plastic surgeons. Plast Reconstr Surg. 1983;72(2):165–9.
58. Mirzabeigi MN, Mericli AF, Ortlip T, Tuma GA, Copit SE, Fox JW, et al. Evaluating the role of postoperative prophylactic antibiotics in primary and secondary breast augmentation: a retrospective review. Aesthet Surg J. 2012;32(1):61–8.
59. Giesecke J, Arnander C. Toxic shock syndrome after augmentation mammaplasty. Ann Plast Surg. 1986;17(6):532–3.
60. Tobin G, Shaw RC, Goodpasture HC. Toxic shock syndrome following breast and nasal surgery. Plast Reconstr Surg. 1987;80(1):111–4.
61. Freedman AM, Jackson IT. Infections in breast implants. Infect Dis Clin N Am. 1989;3(2):275–87.
62. Barnett A, Lavey E, Pearl RM, Vistnes LM. Toxic shock syndrome from an infected breast prosthesis. Ann Plast Surg. 1983;10(5):408–10.
63. Holm C, Mühlbauer W. Toxic shock syndrome in plastic surgery patients: case report and review of the literature. Aesthet Plast Surg. 1998;22(3):180–4.
64. Ablaza VJ, LaTrenta GS. Late infection of a breast prosthesis with Enterococcus avium. Plast Reconstr Surg. 1998;102(1):227–30.
65. Johnson LB, Busuito MJ, Khatib R. Breast implant infection in a cat owner due to Pasteurella multocida. J Infect. 2000;41(1):110–1.
66. Washer LL, Gutowski K. Breast implant infections. Infect Dis Clin N Am. 2012;26(1):111–25.
67. Wu PS, Winocour S, Jacobson SR. Red breast syndrome: a review of available literature. Aesthet Plast Surg. 2015;39(2):227–30.
68. Nguyen TC, Brown AM, Kulber DA, Moliver CL, Kuehnert MJ. The role of endotoxin in sterile inflammation after implanted acellular dermal matrix: red breast syndrome explained? Aesthet Surg J. 2020;40(4):392–9.
69. Cook J, Holmes CJ, Wixtrom R, Newman MI, Pozner J. Characterizing the microbiome of the contracted breast capsule using next generation sequencing. Aesthet Surg J. 2021;41(4):440–7.
70. Fodor L, Ramon Y, Ullmann Y, Eldor L, Peled IJ. Fate of exposed breast implants in augmentation mammoplasty. Ann Plast Surg. 2003;50(5):447–9.

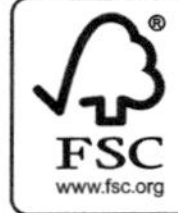